Glomerulonephritis and Nephrotic Syndrome

Edited by Thomas Rath

Published in London, United Kingdom

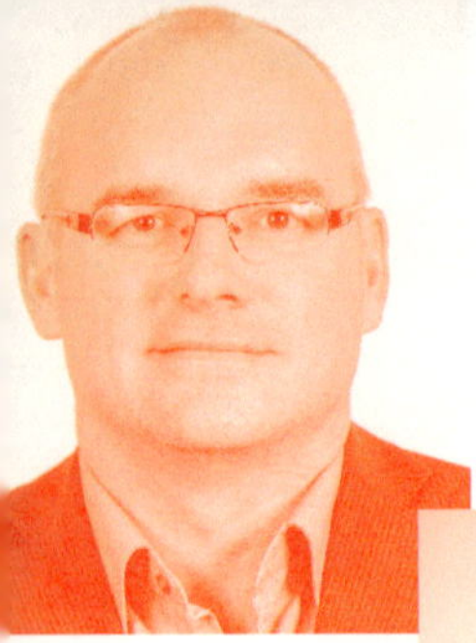
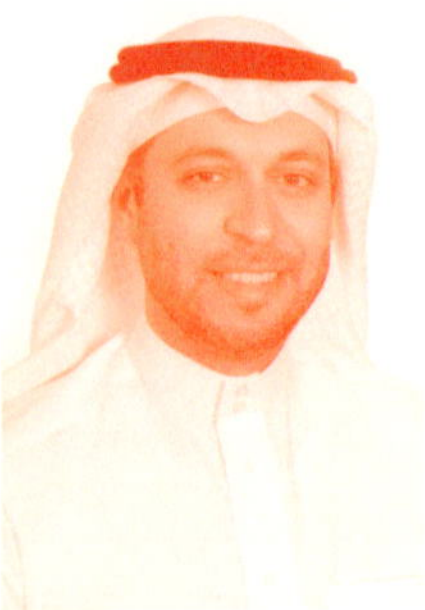
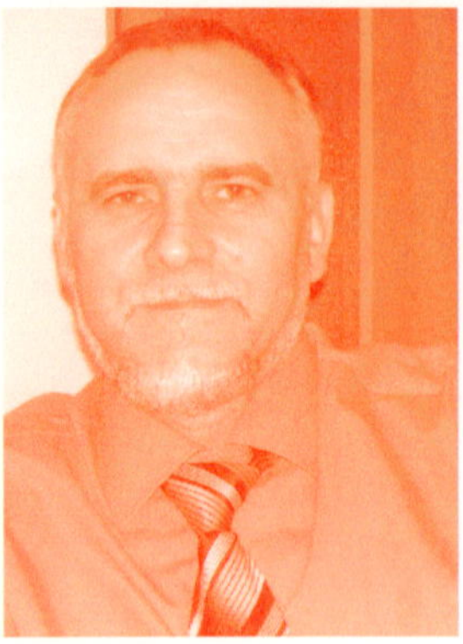
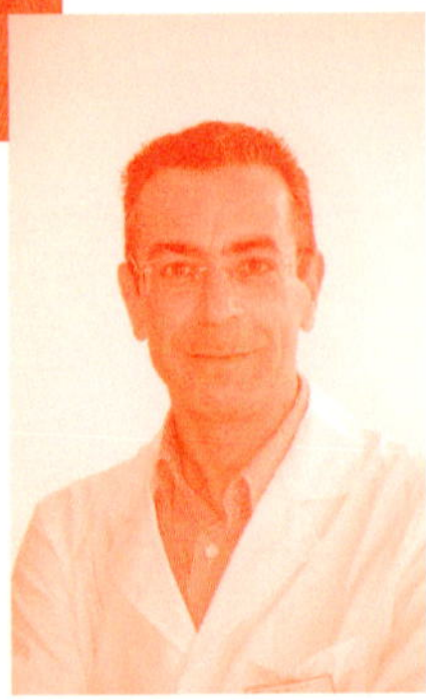
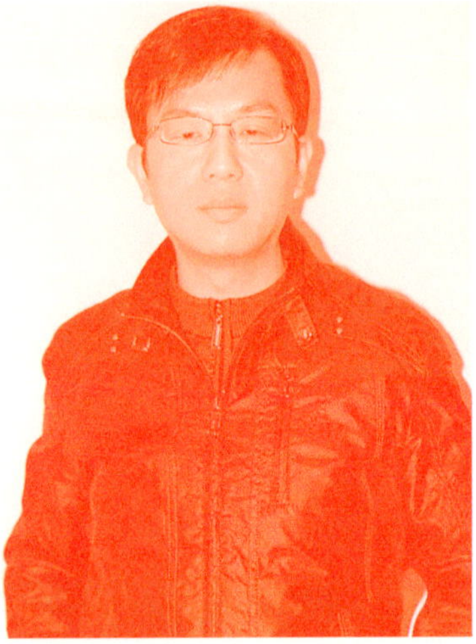
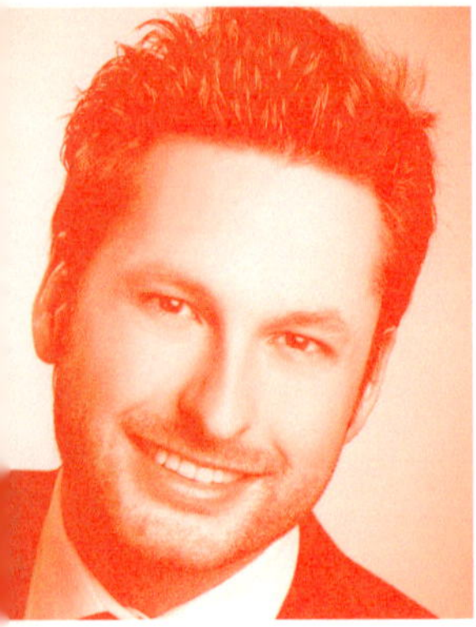
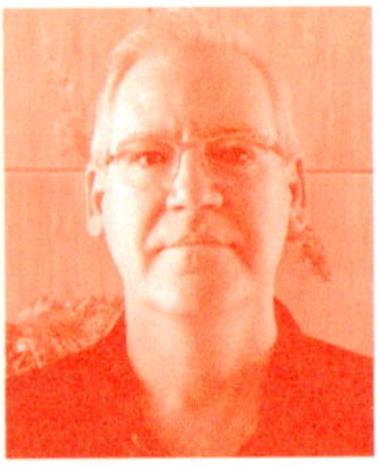

IntechOpen

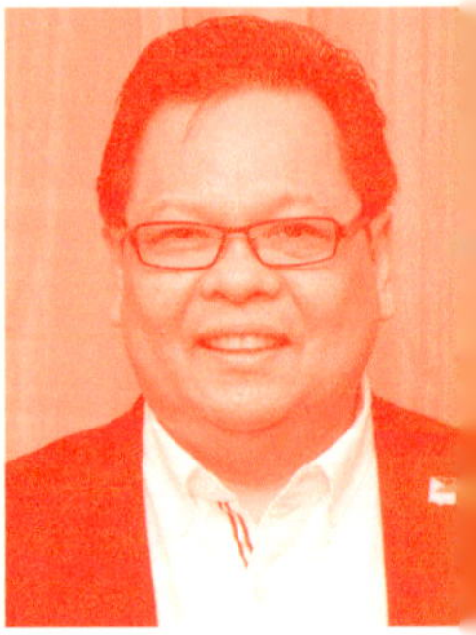
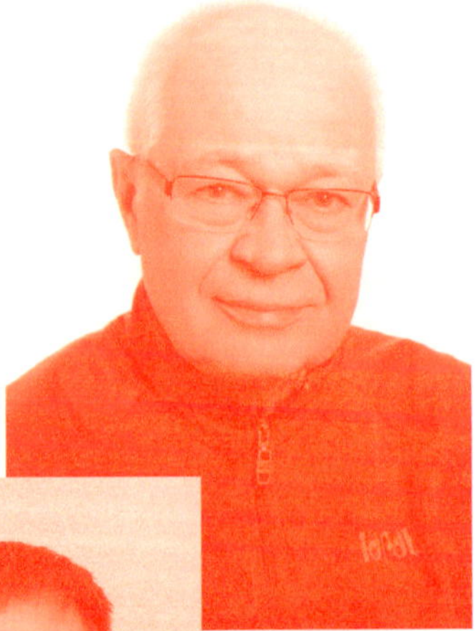
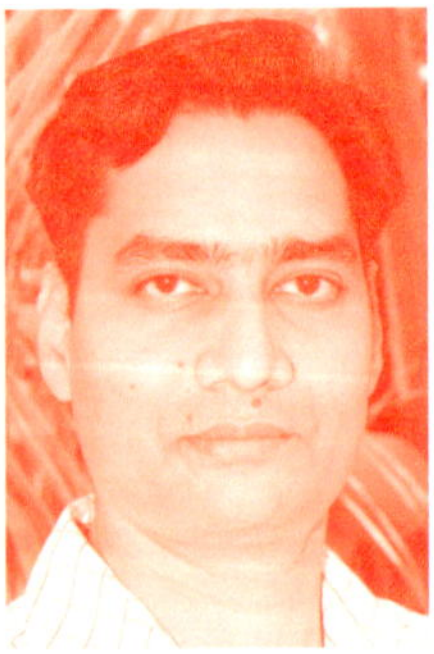
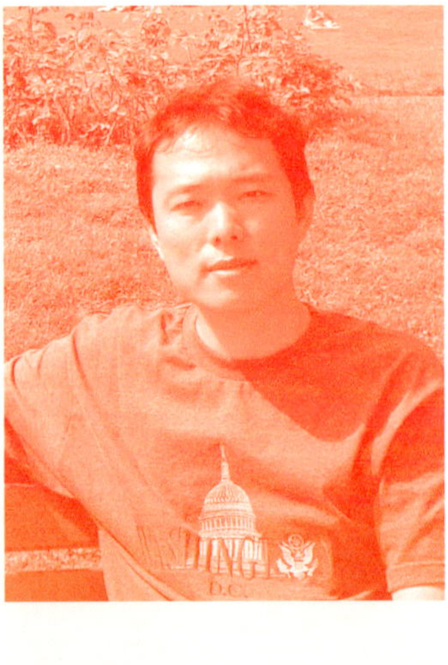
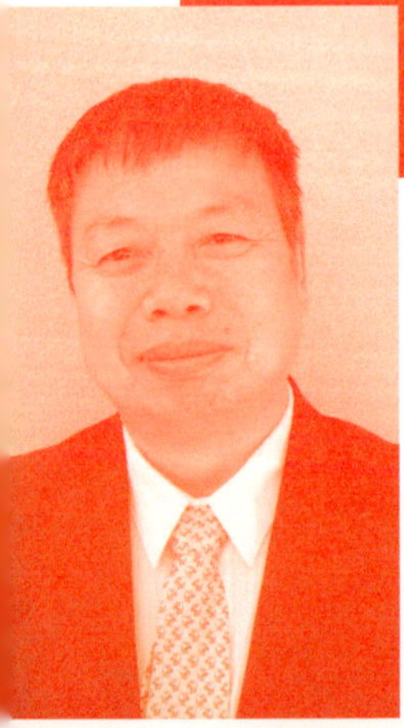
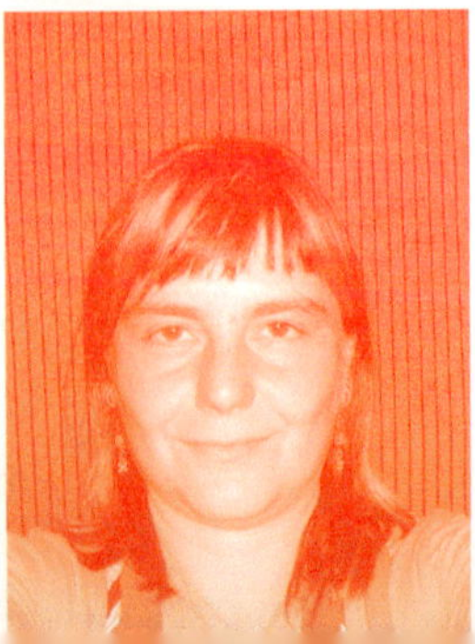

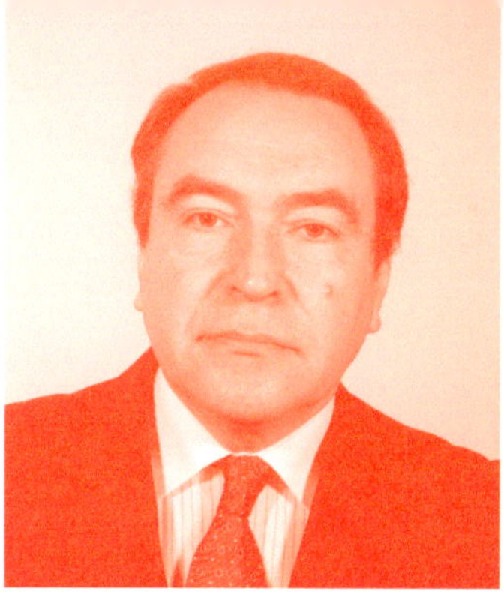

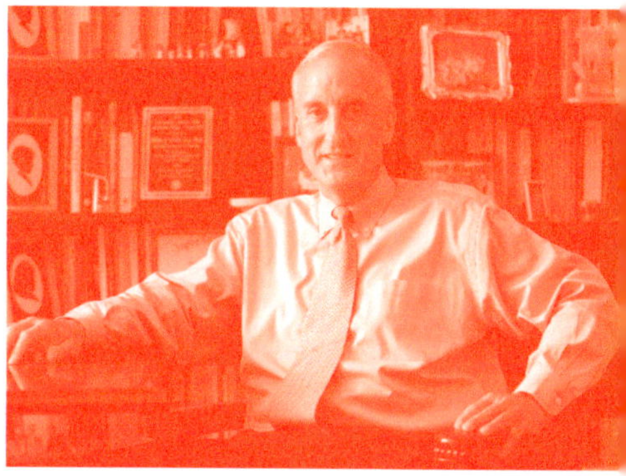

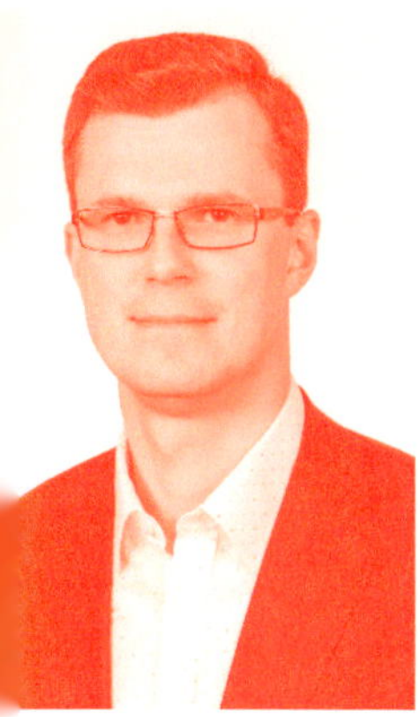

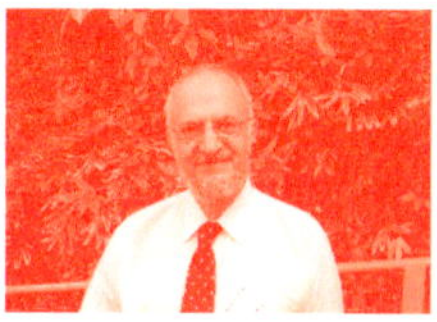

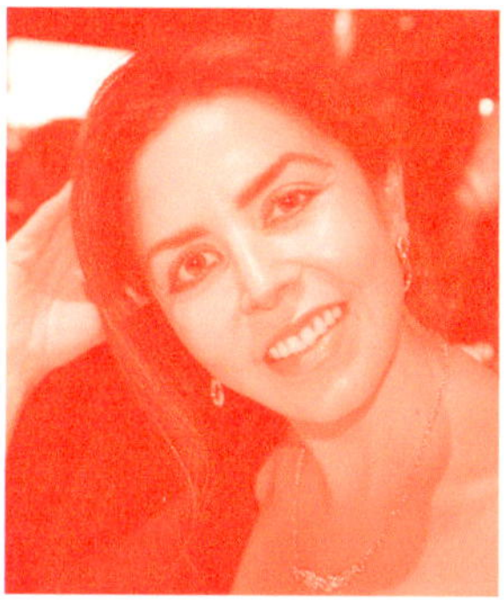

Supporting open minds since 2005

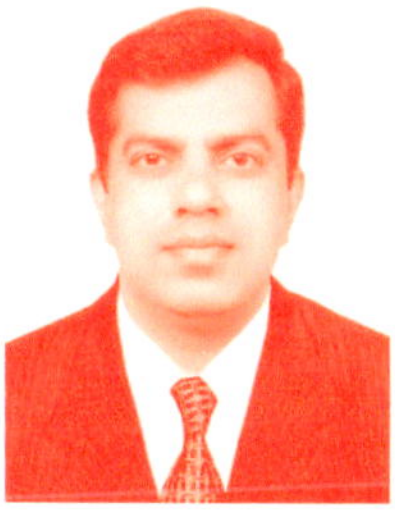

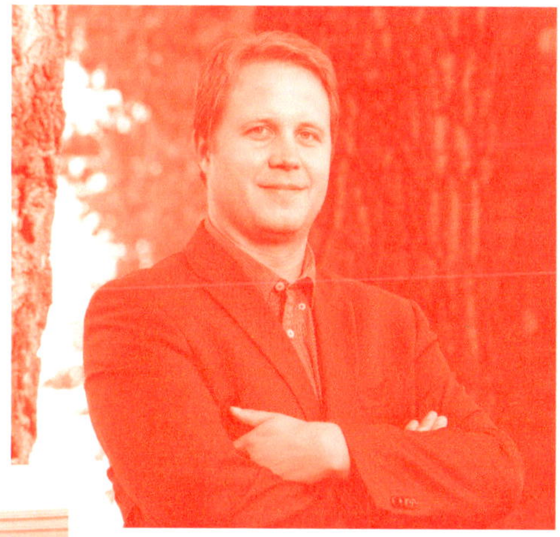

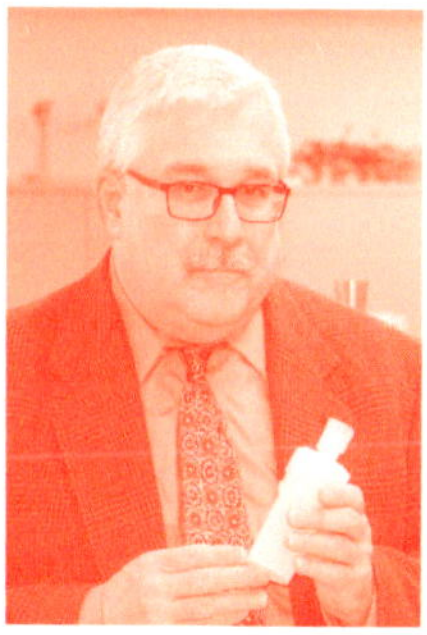

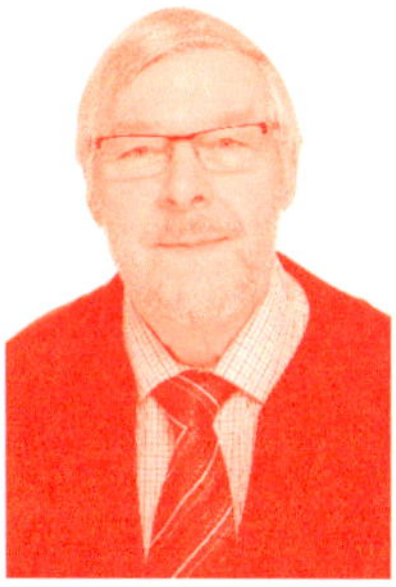

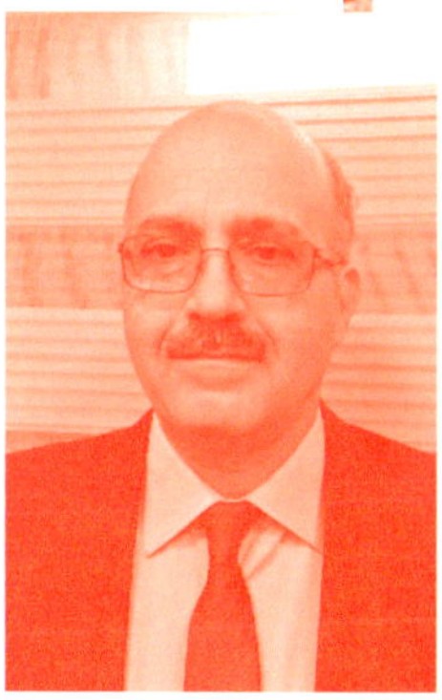

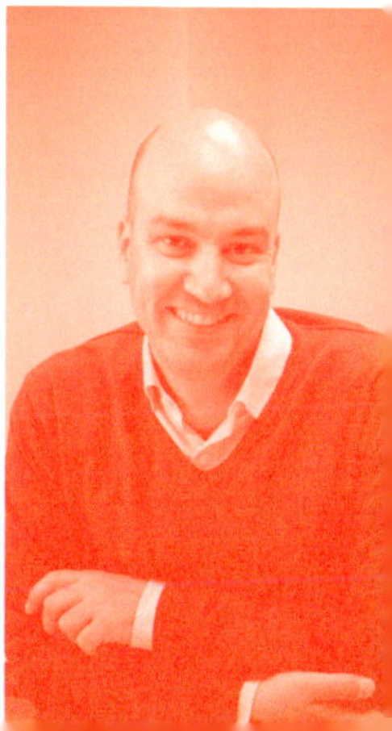

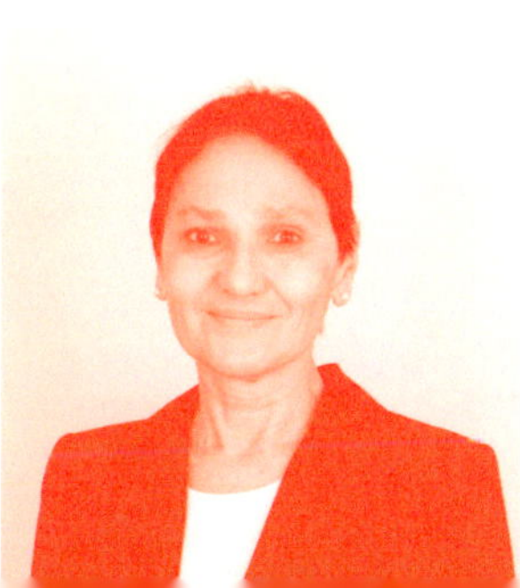

Glomerulonephritis and Nephrotic Syndrome
http://dx.doi.org/10.5772/intechopen.78833
Edited by Thomas Rath

Contributors
Samuel N. Uwaezuoke, Barbara Katharina Geist, María Carmen Prados Soler, María Dolores Del Pino Y Pino, Álvaro Pérez Fernández, Llenalia Gordillo García, María José López Ruiz, César Luis Ramirez-Tortosa, Jorge Enrique Moreno Collazos, Diana Carolina Zona Rubio, David Johnson, Bhadran Bose, Sunil V. Badve, Chen Au Peh, Vivekanand Jha, Maria Stangou, Polyvios Arseniou, Stamatina Stai, Patrick Hamilton, Paul Brenchley, Durga Kanigicherla

First published in London, United Kingdom, 2019 by IntechOpen
IntechOpen is the global imprint of INTECHOPEN LIMITED, registered in England and Wales, registration number: 11086078, 7th floor, 10 Lower Thames Street, London, EC3R 6AF, United Kingdom
Printed in Croatia

British Library Cataloguing-in-Publication Data
A catalogue record for this book is available from the British Library

Additional hard and PDF copies can be obtained from orders@intechopen.com

Glomerulonephritis and Nephrotic Syndrome
Edited by Thomas Rath
p. cm.
Print ISBN 978-1-78984-313-2
Online ISBN 978-1-78984-314-9
eBook (PDF) ISBN 978-1-83962-383-7

For EU product safety concerns:
IN TECH d.o.o., Prolaz Marije Krucifikse Kozulić 3, 51000 Rijeka, Croatia, info@intechopen.com or visit our website at intechopen.com.

Meet the editor

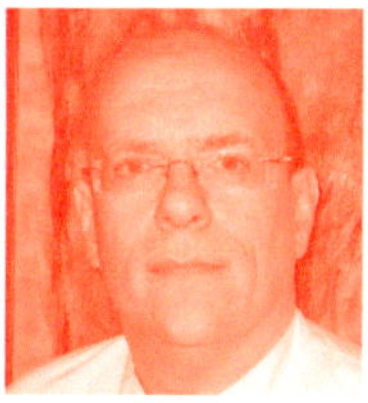

Thomas Rath is a doctor of medicine and specialist in internal medicine, nephrology, hypertension, and infectious diseases. He lives in Kaiserslautern, a city of 100,000 inhabitants in the southwest part of Germany. After completing his studies at the University of Mainz, he became a resident at the Westpfalz-Klinikum in Kaiserslautern, a tertiary care hospital with 1300 hospital beds. There, he is Head of the Department of Nephrology and Transplantation Medicine and also responsible for the outpatient clinic for patients with infectious diseases. He is an active member of many national and international societies. During his scientific career he has published more than 25 papers in peer-reviewed journals and more than 150 abstracts and posters at national and international congresses. He gives lectures at the Technical University of Kaiserslautern on "artificial organ support."

Contents

Preface

Chronic kidney disease (CKD) is a worldwide disease affecting up to 4% of the population with increasing figures also in developing countries. Life expectancy of patients affected by CKD is shortened compared to the overall population and only a minority of the patients reaches end-stage renal disease with the need for dialysis or renal transplantation; death overtakes dialysis. In many cases, glomerulonephritis is the underlying disease leading to kidney failure. One hallmark of glomerulonephritis is proteinuria, which may in its most severe form lead to nephrotic syndrome. Clinically, the syndrome presents with massive proteinuria, hypoalbuminuria, edema, and hyperlipidemia. In children, idiopathic nephrotic syndrome is the commonest manifestation of glomerular disease. Although the genetics of congenital forms are well known to the pediatrician, secondary forms of nephrotic syndrome caused by different types of glomerulonephritis are encountered. The etiopathogenesis of nephrotic syndrome has evolved over several years and theories. Now, podocyte injury is thought to be the keystone in the pathology of different forms of glomerulonephritis associated with massive proteinuria. Therefore, one chapter aims to highlight the mechanisms underlying the pathogenesis of nephrotic syndrome as a podocytopathy, especially in children.

But also in adults, nephrotic syndrome caused by different types of glomerulonephritis occurs. One form of glomerulonephritis of special interest is membranous nephropathy. In non-diabetic Caucasian adults, membranous nephropathy is the leading cause of nephrotic syndrome. There, membranous nephropathy is most often primary (idiopathic) and the remaining is secondary to systemic disease or exposure to infection or drugs. The therapeutic approach reaches from supportive care to immunosuppressive protocols, always trying to minimize proteinuria.

Three chapters of this book focus on membranous nephropathy. There is a fine and concise review of the epidemiology, diagnosis, and treatment of membranous nephropathy, particularly focusing on idiopathic membranous nephropathy. Another chapter strengthens the aspect of membranous nephropathy as an autoimmune disease, aiming to increase our current understanding of autoimmune membranous nephropathy and use it as a basis for the understanding of autoimmune disease in general.

One important clinical aspect in patients with nephrotic syndrome, especially in membranous nephropathy, is increased risk for venous thrombosis. Hypercoagulopathy as a result of the loss of antithrombotic factors such as antithrombin III and plasminogen due to proteinuria, an increased level of factor VIII and fibrinogen, along with increased platelet reactivity have been noted in nephrotic syndrome whatever the cause. However, compared to other conditions that have a similar degree of proteinuria, membranous nephropathy has a higher risk of venous thrombosis and its associated risks.

Interestingly, many patients with membranous nephropathy have circulating antibodies to different podocyte antigens, and immunologic remission (depletion of PLA2R antibodies) often precedes and may predict clinical remission. The use of biomarkers in glomerular diseases is not restricted to membranous nephropathy. Biomarkers provide worthwhile evidence in diagnosis, guide treatment strategies, and give information about prognostic aspects. The importance of several substances and molecules, such as inflammatory cells, autoantibodies, cytokines, chemokines, and growth factors and their role as potential biomarkers, is also described in this book.

Although our knowledge of renal disease has grown, and dialysis treatment is available worldwide, we do not know to what extent low physical activity, uremia, and anemia determine the decrease in functional capacity of patients on dialysis. Therefore, the final chapter of the book will focus on the aspects of rehabilitation in patients with severe kidney disease.

This book comprises a total of seven chapters from authors and researchers from different countries and continents, thus reflecting the worldwide importance of CKD.

We are grateful to all the contributors and experts for the preparation and submission of their stimulating manuscripts. And, last but not least, many thanks go to the team of IntechOpen who gave us the opportunity to publish all these very interesting papers and thoughts in a peer-reviewed Open Access book.

Thomas Rath
Department of Nephrology and Transplantation Medicine,
Westpfalz-Klinikum, Kaiserslautern,
Germany

Section 1

Measuring Kidney Function

Chapter 1

Calculation of GFR via the Slope-Intercept Method in Nuclear Medicine

Barbara Katharina Geist

Abstract

A determination of the glomerular filtration rate (GFR) with high accuracy is of great relevance especially in cases of insufficient kidney function. In nuclear medicine, the standard method is based on blood sample measurements with Cr-51 ethylenediaminetetraacetic acid (Cr-51-EDTA) or Tc-99m diethylene-triamine-pentaacetate (Tc-99m-DTPA), providing very high accuracy and reliability. In particular, the slope-intercept method turned out to be the most appropriate and is therefore routinely used in many hospitals worldwide. For this purpose, blood samples are drawn at certain time points starting 120 minutes after injection, which are then measured together with a standard probe in a gamma counter; based on the results, the GFR calculation is then usually performed automatically with an appropriate software. In this chapter, the mathematical background as well as a step-by-step description of the slope-intercept method is given. In our study, we found that at least three blood samples should be drawn in order to achieve highest quality and reliability. Furthermore, a sample size of at least three blood samples allows an error calculation which provides an estimation of the reliability of the preceding measurement.

Keywords: glomerular filtration rate, slope-intercept method, error calculation, nuclear medicine, Cr-EDTA, Tc-DTPA

1. Introduction

The glomerular filtration rate (GFR) is an important clinical measure for estimating not only the health of the kidneys but also the overall health of a patient, since it is directly proportional to the number of working nephrons. However, an exact determination of the GFR is not simple, and very often, an estimated GFR (eGFR) is calculated from the serum creatinine in the blood [1, 2]. For this, various formulas are available for different purposes [2–4]. Although these methods are convenient, they are not very sensitive, in particular in the case of insufficient kidney function [5].

An approved method for an accurate determination of the GFR was the inulin clearance, because inulin serves as a marker which is filtered by the glomeruli without tubular secretion or reabsorption [6]. Considered as gold standard, this method is time-consuming and needs urine as well as blood sample collection.

In nuclear medicine, several invasive and noninvasive methods are available to calculate the GFR. In principle, radiotracers, i.e., biological markers labeled with a radioactive isotope, are injected into the patient. The behavior of the tracer gives

 IntechOpen

information about the health condition of the organ and can be tracked by the emitted radiation from the labeled isotope. After injection, the radiation and therefore the concentration of the tracer can be measured either from drawn blood samples or with imaging techniques (so-called renal scintigraphy). The latter thus additionally allow a visualization of the anatomical properties of the organ.

To give an example, the very common radio tracer MAG3 (mercaptoacetyl-triglycine, labeled to the gamma emitting isotope Tc-99m), providing excellent image quality, is not filtered in the glomeruli and therefore used with imaging techniques to determine the split renal function and the renal transit [7]. In contrary, the tracers Tc-99m diethylene-triamine-pentaacetate (Tc-99m-DTPA) and Cr-51 ethylenediaminetetraacetic acid (Cr-51-EDTA) are similar to inulin and therefore used to determine the GFR [8].

Cr-51-EDTA is only suitable for blood sample measurements since the physical properties of its labeled isotope Cr-51 do not allow the usage of imaging techniques. Tc-99m-DTPA on the other hand might be used for both blood sample and imaging methods.

For the sake of completeness, it is mentioned that methods are available to estimate the GFR from renal scintigraphy images, based on the accumulation of Tc-99m-DTPA in the kidneys within the first minutes after injection [9]. However, these methods only provide an estimation of the GFR and will therefore not be discussed in this chapter.

The main purpose of this chapter is to introduce the idea and the measurement procedure of the so-called slope-intercept method. In short, an appropriate tracer such as Tc-99m-DTPA or Cr-51-EDTA is injected, and at least two blood samples are taken at certain time points after the injections. The blood samples are then measured in a detector, a so-called gamma counter, in order to determine the emitted radiation, from which the GFR can be calculated. Methods using only one or two blood samples exist, but these are less accurate and error-prone [10]. The most accurate method involves the measurement of at least three blood samples because in this case a determination of the systematic error can be provided which in turn gives information about the reliability of the measurement.

2. Mathematical background

2.1 GFR calculation

For the determination of the GFR from an appropriate tracer, e.g., Tc-99m-DTPA or Cr-51-EDTA, the area under the so-called plasma concentration curve is needed, which is obtained from the drawn blood samples as described in the following.

After injection, the tracer travels through the blood vessels into the kidneys, where it is freely filtered and finally excreted. Assuming that other renal processes of the tracer are negligible, the decrease of the tracer concentration in the blood plasma after certain time points is then a measure for the glomerular filtration. Ideally, starting at 1 hour after injection, every 30 or 60 minutes a blood sample is drawn, in particular in the case of three blood samples at 120, 180, and 240 minutes after injection (see **Figure 1**) [11]. Due to its radioactivity, i.e., its emission of radiation, the tracer concentration in the blood plasma samples can be measured, usually with a gamma counter which allows the measurement of small samples.

The decrease of the tracer concentration in the blood plasma, expressed with a function $P(t)$, follows an exponential decay. This means due to glomerular filtration, the initial tracer concentration in the body (P_0) is decreasing exponentially (time, t) with a certain biological decrease constant L.

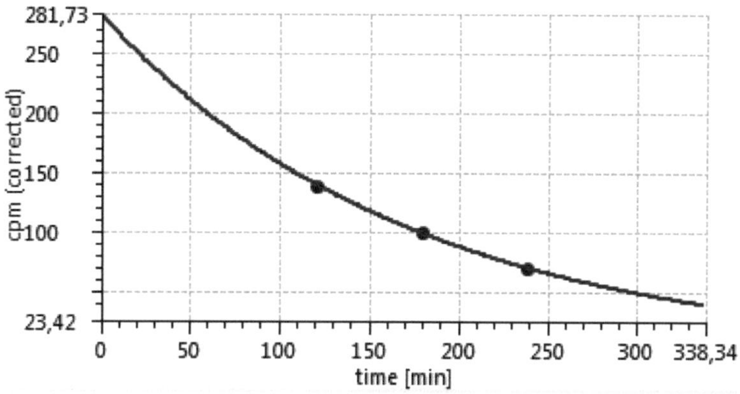

Figure 1.
Measured tracer concentrations of three plasma samples are plotted as dots; an exponential curve (see Eq. (1)) was fitted through the data points (line). The abscissa gives the time in minutes after injection of the tracer.

$$P(t) = P_0 \cdot e^{-L \cdot t} \tag{1}$$

The area A under this curve obviously is

$$A = \frac{P_0}{L} \tag{2}$$

The curve $P(t)$ is obtained by fitting the measured blood plasma samples with the exponential function from Eq. (1) (see **Figure 1**), e.g., with a least squares algorithm. The fit parameters are the values P_0 (the "intercept") and L (the "slope"), which are then used to calculate A.

Another information needed for the GFR calculation is the applied dose to the patient. While the syringe with the tracer is measured in an activimeter (or a comparable detector) before injection, the blood samples, showing considerably less radioactivity, are measured in a very different device (gamma counter). In order to connect the measurements of both devices, a so-called standard (a small amount of the tracer) must be prepared, which is then measured in both devices. The ratio of these two measurements is used to convert the injected dose measured in the activimeter to the units of the gamma counter. The converted applied dose D therefore can be written as

$$D = Act_{Syringe} \cdot \frac{Act_{Std}}{GC_{Std}} \tag{3}$$

with $Act_{Syringe}$ as measured syringe activity before application and Act_{Std} as standard activity in the activimeter and GC_{Std} as measured standard activity in the gamma counter.

The GFR can then be expressed as the converted total dose applied to the patient, D, divided by the area under the plasma concentration curve [11]

$$GFR = \frac{D \cdot V}{A} \tag{4}$$

with V as the dilution of the standard (usually around 500, see Section 3). Therefore, using Eqs. (2) and (3), the GFR can be written as

$$GFR = Act_{Syringe} \cdot \frac{Act_{Std}}{GC_{Std}} \cdot V \cdot \frac{L}{P_0} \tag{5}$$

2.2 Corrections

2.2.1 AUC correction

Due to underlying biological processes, the plasma concentration curve $P(t)$ appears not as a perfect exponential decay in particular in the beginning, leading to a wrong area under the curve (AUC). This can be solved by fitting the curve with multiple exponential curves, which would need much more blood samples. Another option is to start blood sample withdrawal after 120 minutes, i.e., after initial renal processes, using a simple AUC correction formula. Several formulas for adults and children are provided [11–14]. The Brochner-Mortensen correction is recommended [11, 15]:

For adults

$$GFR_{corr} = 0.9908 \cdot GFR - 0.001218 \cdot GFR^2$$

For children

$$GFR_{corr} = 1.01 \cdot GFR - 0.0017 \cdot GFR^2$$

2.2.2 Radioactive decay correction

Furthermore, both tracers not only have a biological half-life due to their glomerular clearance but also a physical half-life due to the radioactivity of their labeled isotopes. Consequently, the tracer concentration in the blood samples not only decreases due to the biological clearance but virtually also due to the physical loss of decayed isotopes which are labeled to the tracer.

Keeping in mind that the blood samples for the GFR determination with the slope-intercept method must be drawn 3 or even more hours after injection and the half-life of the isotope is not infinite, the physical half-life of the isotope might lead to a significant loss of tracer concentration due to its radioactivity (and not due to glomerular filtration). Ideally, the physical half-life of the corresponding isotope therefore should be very high in order to minimize the concentration loss due to radioactivity. This issue is illustrated in **Figure 2**.

In case of Cr-51-EDTA, the physical half-life of Cr-51 is 27.7 days. Assuming that, starting with injection, the blood sample withdrawing takes 4 hours, one can easily calculate that the virtual loss of tracer concentration due to its radioactivity during this time interval is about 1%. The radioactivity of Cr-51 therefore can be considered as negligible and the tracer can be treated as physically stable (see **Figure 2**).

On the other hand, the isotope Tc-99m from the tracer Tc-99m-DTPA has a physical half-life of about 6 hours; the concentration loss during a time period of 4 hours is not negligible anymore. As illustrated in **Figure 2**, measured values of drawn sample appear with a significantly lower measured concentration value due to the radioactive decay of Tc-99m; in this example, the calculated GFR would be falsely overstated by 20%. Thus, measurements with Tc-99m-DTPA must be corrected for the physical half-life of Tc-99m.

2.2.3 Background correction

Another important issue is the unavoidable measurement of unintended radioactivity. First, the remaining radioactivity in the syringe after injection must be measured and subtracted from the applied dose. Furthermore, both activimeter and

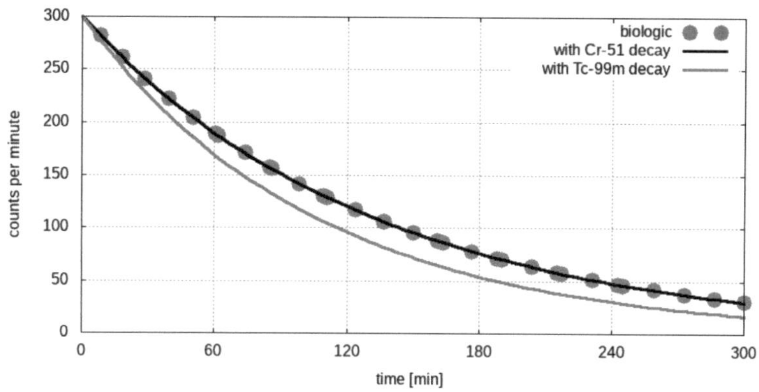

Figure 2.
Exponential decrease due to glomerular filtration with a typical half-life of 90 minutes (gray dots). Due to radioactive decay, real obtained curves are shown as black line in the case of Cr-51 and as gray line in the case of Tc-99m.

gamma counter continuously measure background radiation which must be subtracted from all measured values.

2.2.4 BSA correction

Since the GFR varies with the body surface area (BSA), it usually is presented as pure value but also corrected for the body surface area (BSA-GFR), normalized to the "standard man" (body surface 1.73 m^2). Several formalisms are available to estimate the body surface area for adults and children [16–20].

2.3 Error calculation

In clinical routine, irregularities during the measurement process, inadvertence, radioactive contamination, and other so-called systematic errors might lead to inaccurate results. Statistical (random) errors from the activimeter and gamma counter measurements are assumed to be negligible [10].

To estimate these systematic errors, the error of the area under the tracer concentration curve A (Eq. (2)) can be calculated after the fitting procedure [10], provided at least three blood samples have been taken. According to the Gaussian error propagation law, the errors of L and P_0 need to be calculated in order to obtain the error of A:

$$s_A = \sqrt{\left(\frac{s_{P0}}{L}\right)^2 + \left(\frac{s_L \cdot P_0}{L^2}\right)^2} \tag{6}$$

with s_A as error of the area under the curve A, s_{P0} as error of P_0, and s_L as error of L. This problem can be solved analytically, leading to

$$s_L = \sqrt{n \cdot \frac{1}{n-2} \cdot \frac{\sum (\ln P_0 - Lt_i - lnP(t_i))^2}{n \sum t_i^2 - (\sum t_i)^2}} \tag{7}$$

$$s_{P0} = P_0 \cdot \sqrt{\sum t_i{}^2 \cdot \frac{1}{n-2} \cdot \frac{\sum (\ln P_0 - Lt_i - lnP(t_i))^2}{n \sum t_i^2 - (\sum t_i)^2}} \tag{8}$$

with t_i as time interval after injection.

Under the assumption that random errors are negligible, s_A represents the error of the calculated GFR. Although errors of <10% are considered insignificant, high errors allow to identify irregularities and re-evaluate the results.

3. Measurement

3.1 Preparation

A standard is prepared, i.e., 1 ml of the used tracer is filled in an appropriate holder. Both the standard and the full syringe are measured in the activimeter. The empty syringe must also be measured after application in order to subtract the remaining activity from the measured value before application. In Eq. (3), this delivers the values $Act_{Syringe}$ and Act_{Std}.

3.2 Blood sample measurement

At least three blood samples are taken, starting at 120 minutes after injection, with an interval of 1 hour. The exact time period between injection and blood sample withdrawal needs to be recorded in order to minimize errors.

The standard usually needs to be diluted, e.g., by a factor of around 500. Around 1 ml is transferred into holders appropriate for the gamma counter. After separating blood plasma from hematocrit, 1 ml of each plasma sample is also transferred into holders for the gamma counter; all probes are measured. This gives the value GC_{Std} as well as all necessary data points to obtain the plasma concentration curve $P(t)$ (Eq. (1)).

3.3 GFR calculation procedure

Before starting any calculations, all measured values need to be corrected for background. Note that in case of Tc-99m-DTPA, values need to be corrected for radioactive decay. The measured data points are fitted with an exponential function (Eq. (1)) to obtain the plasma concentration curve function $P(t)$ and from this P_0 and L, which are needed to calculate the GFR (Eq. (5)).

If possible, i.e., if more than two blood samples have been drawn, the error is calculated according to Eq. (6). Furthermore, AUC correction and BSA correction are applied to the final GFR result.

4. Comparison of different blood sample methods

There are several methods allowing an estimation of the GFR from only one blood sample [21–24]. Although these methods are from high convenience for the routine and the patients, they are not recommended for low GFRs [11] and show significant deviations to the slope-intercept method [10].

The slope-intercept method with blood samples drawn after 120 minutes after injection is suggested to be the best compromise between accuracy and simplicity; it furthermore is a repeatable and reliable method [10, 11, 25, 26]. Since an error calculation helps in identifying errors in the measurement process such as radioactive contamination or irregularities in the routine, the slope-intercept method with three blood samples appears ideal.

5. Conclusions

The slope-intercept method is based on several blood samples and an accurate calculation procedure including corrections and error estimation. In particular in case of low GFRs, this method is the best compromise between the effort for the clinical routine, patients comfort, and accuracy.

Appendices and nomenclature

Abbreviations

AUC	area under the curve
BSA	body surface area
GFR	glomerular filtration rate

Nomenclature

Tc-99m-DTPA	Tc-99m diethylene-triamine-pentaacetate
Cr-51-EDTA	Cr-51ethylenediaminetetraacetic acid

Author details

Barbara Katharina Geist
Department of Biomedical Imaging and Image-Guided Therapy, Division of Nuclear Medicine, Vienna, Austria

*Address all correspondence to: barbara.geist@meduniwien.ac.at

References

[1] National Kidney Foundation. K/ DOQI clinical practice guidelines for chronic kidney disease: Evaluation, classification, and stratification. American Journal of Kidney Diseases. 2002;**39**:S1-S266

[2] Levey AS, Stevens LA, Schmid CH, Zhang Y, Castro AF, Feldman HI, et al. New equation to estimate glomerular filtration rate. Annals of Internal Medicine. 2009;**150**:604-612

[3] Levey AS, Bosch JP, Lewis JB, Greene T, Rogers N, Roth D. A more accurate method to estimate glomerular filtration rate from serum creatinine: A new prediction equation. Modification of diet in renal disease study group. Annals of Internal Medicine. 1999;**130**:461-470

[4] Cockcroft DW, Gault MH. Prediction of creatinine clearance from serum creatinine. Nephron. 1976;**16**: 31-41

[5] Chew DJ, DiBartola S. Diagnosis and pathophysiology of renal disease. In: Ettinger SJ, editor. Textbook of Veterinary Internal Medicine. Philadelphia: WB Saunders; 1989. pp. 1893-1962

[6] Walser M, Davidson DG, Orloff J. The renal clearance of alkali-stable inulin. The Journal of Clinical Investigation;**34**:1520-1523

[7] Al-NahhasRafaqat AA, Jafri RA, Britton KE, Solanki K, Bomanji J, Mather S, et al. Clinical experience with 99mTc-MAG3, mercaptoacetyl-triglycine, and a comparison with 99mTc-DTPA. European Journal of Nuclear Medicine. 1988;**14**:453

[8] Daniel GB, Mitchell SK, Mawby D, Sackman JE, Schmidt D. Renal nuclear medicine: A review. Veterinary Radiology & Ultrasound. 1999;**40**(6): 572-587

[9] Gates GF. Glomerular filtration rate: Estimation from fractional renal accumulation of 99mTc-DTPA. American Journal of Roentgenology. 1982;**138**:565-570

[10] Geist BK, Diemling M, Staudenherz A. Glomerular filtration rate and error calculation based on the slope-intercept method with Chromium-51 ethylenediaminetetraacetic acid via a new clinical software: GFRcalc. Medical Principles and Practice. 2016;**25**(4): 368-373

[11] Fleming JS, Zivanovic MA, Blake GM, Burniston M, Cosgriff PS. Guidelines for the measurement of glomerular filtration rate using plasma sampling. Nuclear Medicine Communications. 2004;**25**:759-769

[12] Brochner-Mortensen J. A simple method for the determination of glomerular filtration rate. Scandinavian Journal of Clinical and Laboratory Investigation. 1972;**30**:271-274

[13] Brochner-Mortensen J, Haahr J, Christoffersen J. A simple method for accurate assessment of the glomerular filtration rate in children. Scandinavian Journal of Clinical and Laboratory Investigation. 1974;**33**:140-143

[14] Jodal L, Brochner-Mortensen J. Reassessment of a classical single injection 51Cr-EDTA clearance method for determination of renal function in children and adults. Part I: Analytically correct relationship between total and one-pool clearance. Scandinavian Journal of Clinical and Laboratory Investigation. 2009;**69**:305-313

[15] Murray AW, Barnfield MC, Waller ML, Telford T, Peter AM. Assessment of

glomerular filtration rate measurement with plasma sampling: A technical review. Journal of Nuclear Medicine Technology. 2013;**41**(2):67-75

[16] Mosteller RD. Simplified calculation of body-surface area. The New England Journal of Medicine. 1987;**317**:1098-1098

[17] DuBois D, EF DB. A formula to estimate the approximate surface area if height and weight be known. Archives of Internal Medicine. 1916;**17**:863-871

[18] Haycock GB, Schwartz GJ, Wisotsky DH. Geometric method for measuring body surface area: A height-weight formula validated in infants, children and adults. The Journal of Pediatrics. 1978;**93**:62-66

[19] Gehan EA, George SL. Estimation of human body surface area from height and weight. Cancer Chemotherapy Reports. 1970;**54**:225-235

[20] Boyd E. The Growth of the Surface Area of the Human Body. Minneapolis: University of Minnesota Press; 1935

[21] Russell CD, Bischoff PG, Kontzen FN, Rowell KL, Yester MV, Lloyd KL, et al. Measurement of glomerular filtration rate: Single injection plasma clearance method without urine collection. Journal of Nuclear Medicine. 1985;**26**:1243-1247

[22] Watson WS. A simple method of estimating glomerular filtration rate. European Journal of Nuclear Medicine. 1992;**19**:827-827

[23] Ham HR, Piepsz A. Estimation of glomerular filtration rate in infants and in children using a single-plasma method. Journal of Nuclear Medicine. 1991;**32**:1294-1297

[24] Hamilton D, Miola UJ. Body surface correction in single-sample methods of glomerular filtration rate estimation. Nuclear Medicine Communications. 1999;**20**:273-278

[25] Chantler C, Baratt TM. Estimation of glomerular filtration Raten from plasma clearance of 51-chromium Edetic acid. Archives of Disease in Childhood. 1972;**47**:613-617

[26] Bird NJ, Peters C, Robert Michell A, Michael Peters A. Comparison of GFR measurements assessed from single versus multiple samples. American Journal of Kidney Diseases. 2009;**54**:278-288

Chapter 2

Biomarkers in Renal Vasculitis

Polyvios Arseniou, Stamatia Stai and Maria Stangou

Abstract

The use of biomarkers in glomerular diseases has been subject of investigation during the last decades, as it can provide worthwhile evidence in diagnosis, but also, it can guide treatment and give information about prognosis and response. Renal biopsy is still the compulsory technique to establish diagnosis, and also to offer information about the severity of renal damage. However, as an invasive method, it cannot be regularly performed during follow up, so the need to find and establish measurement of molecules, easily collected, which are associated with disease pathogenesis and predict renal function outcome seems very attractive to nephrologists. The renal complications of systemic vasculitis are very important for the outcome of the disease, and several substances and molecules, such as inflammatory cells, autoantibodies, cytokines, chemokines and growth factors are produced and may serve as biomarkers to provide useful information for diagnosis, follow up of the disease.

Keywords: vasculitis, biomarkers, cytokines, growth factors, outcome

1. Introduction

The classical presentation of a primary or secondary glomerular disease (GD) is the triad of microscopic hematuria, proteinuria and impaired renal function.

A patient who presents with microhematuria, 2 g of proteinuria and a GRF of around 35 ml/min is possible to have IgAN, focal segmental sclerosis (FSGS) or membranous nephropathy (MN) or focal necrotising glomerulonephritis, due to vasculitis, and the diagnosis will be established with renal biopsy, which is the typical and standard method in diagnosing GN.

However, renal biopsy is an invasive method, which is usually mandatory for diagnosis, but, carrying the probability of complications, it cannot be repeated regularly during follow up. This is the reason, why the need to find and apply biomarkers that could help in diagnosis and follow up of the GNs is imperative.

2. Biomarkers: which are the characteristics of an ideal biomarker?

The precise characteristics of an ideal biomarker depend upon the disease of investigation, but certain features are considered as important, and are depicted in **Table 1**.

Primary and secondary GDs have some unique advantages; first of all kidneys produce urine, and urine are easy to collect in order to repeat measurements during follow up, but also excreted molecules in the urine represent histological changes in the kidneys. Nevertheless, kidneys are highly perfused organs, meaning that any

IntechOpen

1.	High sensitivity
2.	High specificity
3.	Biological plausibility
4.	Associated with pathogenic mechanisms
5.	Prognosis and response to treatment
6.	Biomarker sources should be easily available

Table 1.
Specific characteristics, an ideal biomarker should carry.

substances in the serum may have a direct effect on them. On the other hand, there are major disadvantages. Pathogenesis of GDs, especially of vasculitis affecting kidneys, is not a simple issue, it is complicated and in most cases not completely identified. Histological lesions are the result of different synergistic or counteracting pathways, which lead to proliferation, inflammation and fibrosis. In addition, the same molecule will not have the same effect in all glomerular diseases [1–5].

All the above mean that all the information provided by kidney biopsy cannot be easily substituted by one biomarker, and the question that comes up is: do the biomarkers have something to offer which is beyond the renal biopsy results and beyond the classical approach of glomerular diseases, including estimation of renal function impairment, degree of proteinuria, microhematuria and active urine sediment, or do they just correlate with these parameters and reflect renal damage?

In the present chapter, we are going to describe biomarkers involved in pathogenesis and outcome of systemic vasculitis affecting the kidneys, and we shall investigate possible advantage instead of using classical parameters.

3. ANCA-associated vasculitides

ANCA-associated vasculitides (AAV) are a group of systemic pauci-immune diseases, characterized by inflammatory necrosis of the small vessels (arterioles, capillaries and venules) and the presence of antineutrophil cytoplasmic antibodies (ANCA) [6–11]. There are four clinical and pathological phenotypes of AAV: granulomatosis with polyangiitis (GPA, formerly known as Wegener's granulomatosis), eosinophilic granulomatosis with polyangiitis (EGPA, also known as Churg-Strauss syndrome), microscopic polyangiitis (MPA) and, finally, renal limited vasculitis (RLV), also known as idiopathic rapidly progressive glomerulonephritis (RPGN) [9, 11]. Contrary to other small-vessel vasculitides, which are immune-complex-mediated, in AAV there is no significant immunoglobulin deposition [6, 9–11].

4. ANCA

ANCA are IgG autoantibodies directed against proteinase 3 (PR3-ANCA), expressed in neutrophil granules, and myeloperoxidase (MPO-ANCA), expressed in monocyte lysosomes. PR3 and MPO are also expressed in the neutrophil extracellular traps (NET), localized to inflammatory lesions within the affected organs [6–11]. Because of their immunofluorescence pattern, PR3-ANCA are also described as cytoplasmic ANCA (c-ANCA), whereas MPO-ANCA are referred to as perinuclear ANCA (p-ANCA) [5, 9–11]. Indirect immunofluorescence and enzyme-linked immunosorbent assay (ELISA) methods are used to detect ANCA in the serum of patients [9, 11]. The type of ANCA (PR3-ANCA or MPO-ANCA) defines the serotype of the AAV [8, 11].

There is a correlation between the serotype and the phenotype of AAV. PR3-ANCA are most common (75%) in patients with GPA and least common (5%) in patients with EGPA. MPO-ANCA occur more frequently in patients with RLV (70%), while they appear in 60% of patients with EGPA and 50% of patients with MPA. The occurrence of seronegativity is 5 and 30% in GPA and EGPA, respectively, and 10% in MPO and RLV [9]. ANCA-positive patients present either PR3-ANCA or MPO-ANCA, whereas the occurrence of both ANCA in the same individual is extremely rare and related to infection-induced or drug-mediated vasculitis [5, 9–11].

However, autoantibodies against different antigenic targets, such as lysosome-associated membrane protein-2 (LAMP-2), plasminogen, moesin, have been demonstrated recently, and they were related to different precipitating causes, as well as different disease presentation and severity. Specifically, anti-LAMP-2 antibodies have been found in most patients with RLV linked to *E. coli* urinary tract infection (UTI), suggesting that molecular mimicking mechanisms may be responsible for the formation of antibodies [6–10].

5. Pathogenesis

PR3 and MPO antigens are presented by autoreactive antigen-presenting B cells to autoreactive T cells, thus stimulating their activation and polarization, with the formation of pro-inflammatory Th1, Th2 and Th17 cells. In that environment, T cells activate B cells, promoting the formation of ANCA. Autoreactivity of B and T cells is presented in patients with genetic susceptibility, as shown by correlation of the disease with specific HLA gene loci, while both SNP in certain genes and epigenetic factors are associated with increased antigenic expression in neutrophils and monocytes. That increased expression of PR3 on the monocyte cell surface causes macrophage activation, while binding of MPO-ANCA promotes the release of pro-inflammatory cytokines, such as IL-1β, IL-6 and IL-8. On the other side, increased PR3 expression on the neutrophil surface, in patients with GPA, promotes diminished macrophage phagocytosis of neutrophils that have undergone apoptosis, leading to uncontrolled necrosis and release of more antigens and pro-inflammatory cytokines, including IL-6, IL-8 and TNF-α, which further amplify the previous pathological immune mechanism [6–11].

The involvement of immune cells in pathogenesis of AAV, through impaired immune tolerance and balance between immune response and immune regulation is crucial. As mentioned, B cells are responsible for antigen presentation and antibody production, but also for cytokine production and activation of T cells. That is why rituximab, a chimeric monoclonal anti-CD20 antibody, is successfully administered as therapy for AAV. Besides that, regulating B cells, which act suppressing immune response, are found numerically normal, but with impaired function. This also applies for regulating T cells, while, on the contrary, effector T cells are found infiltrating affected tissues, alongside with macrophages, neutrophils and monocytes. These cells are responsible for direct tissue damage, releasing reacting oxygen species. Neutrophils, specifically, appear to be the main participating cell in vessel damage, via the respiratory burst and the release of proteolytic enzymes and NET [6–11].

There are recent data from animal and patient studies suggesting that the complement is also involved in AAV. Altered levels of C3, C4, and CH50 are found in some patients during presentation and are associated with adverse outcome. Moreover, C5a and its receptor are implicated in neutrophil activation, thus establishing the alternative compliment pathway as a promoting disease factor and a possible therapeutic target [6–11].

As far as genetic susceptibility is concerned, genome-wide association studies (GWAS) have documented a close relation between the phenotype and serotype of AAV and specific HLA gene loci. In detail, studies on Northern European and American populations have shown that GPA and PR3-ANCA are strongly associated with HLA-DP loci (with HLA-DP 0401 being associated with PR3-ANCA vasculitis and recurrence of disease, regardless of phenotype or serotype), while MPO-ANCA are related to HLA-DQ loci. HLA-DR B1501 is associated with AAV presentation in African American patients and HLA-DR B4 with EGPA. Besides HLA genes, SNP in genes PRTN3, coding for PR3, and SERPINA1, coding for a1-antitrypsin (A1AT), a protein regulating PR3, are associated with the formation of PR3-ANCA, while SNP in gene PTPN22, coding for a protein tyrosine phosphatase, regulating B and T cell receptor-mediated cell activation, is implicated in the dysregulation of immune response [6–11].

6. Clinical presentation

AAV is, as mentioned before, a necrotizing inflammation of the small vessels. Therefore, it is considered a systemic disorder, affecting all tissues and organs. The clinical presentation depends on the activity and the chronicity of the disease and the specific system involvement and determines, together with the pathology, the phenotype of the disease [9].

The onset of the disease may be accompanied by non-specific systemic symptoms, such as fever, fatigue, malaise, anorexia, weight loss, arthralgia and myalgia. These symptoms, reminiscent of flu-like illness, may precede weeks or even months before the occurrence of specific systemic manifestations [9, 12].

Renal involvement is the most significant and severe of AAV clinical presentation. It affects almost every patient with MPA (90%) and GPA (80%), but less than half of the patients with EGPA (45%). The most common presentation is with RPGN, thus featuring typically microscopic or gross hematuria, subnephrotic proteinuria, hypertension, edema and, finally, renal failure, while examination of the urine reveals active urinary sediment, with dysmorphic red blood cells and red blood cell casts. Another presentation, common to patients with MPO-ANCA, is indolent glomerulonephritis, featuring a more chronic presence of microscopic hematuria and a slower decline of renal function. Interestingly, 5% of the patients with ANCA vasculitis (mostly MPO-ANCA) are also positive for anti-glomerular base membrane (anti-GBM) antibodies, suggesting concomitant glomerular lesions of AAV and anti-GBM disease. Renal involvement is the only manifestation of RLV [9, 11, 12].

Lower respiratory system involvement is more frequent in GPA (90%) and EGPA (70%) and less frequent in MPA (50%). Pulmonary manifestations vary from transient infiltration of the alveoli to severe pulmonary hemorrhage. Clinical, laboratory and imaging findings include dyspnea, cough, hemoptysis, acid-base balance and blood gases disorder, lung functional tests disorder, as well as radiological ground-glass pattern, with nodules and diffuse infiltrates [9, 11, 12].

Upper respiratory system is also involved in the clinical presentation, concerning mostly patients with GPA (90%), but also half of the patients with EGPA and 35% of the patients with MPA. Patients present sinusitis, rhinitis, ocular inflammatory disorders, such as episcleritis, necrosis and perforation of the nasal septum and subglottic stenosis. Interestingly, EGPA, is less associated with RPGN and pulmonary hemorrhage and is characterized by a prodromal phase of atopic manifestations, asthma and allergic rhinitis, followed by an eosinophilic phase of increased eosinophil counts in the blood and eosinophilic perfusion of affected tissues, before evolving to active vasculitis [9, 11, 12].

Involvement of the central and peripheral nervous system accompanies 70% of patients with EGPA, 50% of patients with GPA and 30% of patients with MPA and manifests usually as mononeuritis multiplex, while the inflammation of the meninges is less frequent [9, 11, 12].

Cardiovascular involvement, mainly in ANCA-negative EGPA patients, presents as endocarditis, pericarditis or myocarditis, hypokinesis of the ventricles arrhythmias, such as atrioventricular blocks, and, lastly, as acute myocardial infarction [9, 11, 12].

Gastrointestinal involvement, affecting half of the patients with AAV, presents as an acute abdomen, with abdominal pain, hematochezia and sometimes even perforation, due to mesenterial ischemia and ulceration [9, 12].

Finally, AAV present with a plethora of cutaneous lesion, such as purpura, petechiae, ecchymoses, ulcers, nodules and more [9].

7. Renal pathology

Renal biopsy is the gold standard for the diagnosis of renal disease, and this also applies for AAV. The classical histopathological feature in renal biopsy of AAV patients

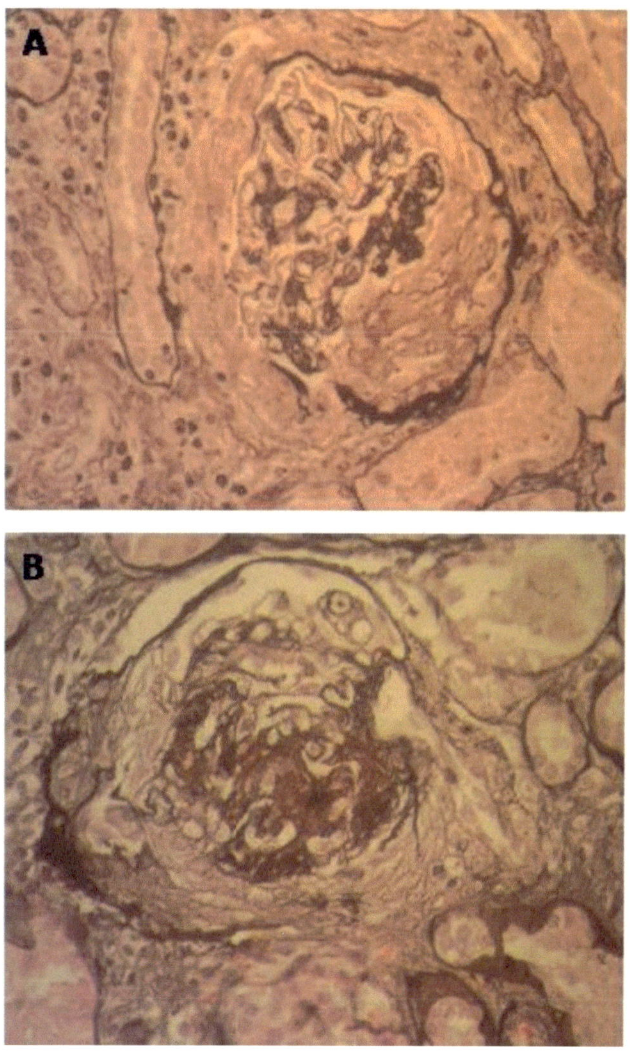

Figure 1.
Histology of renal involvement in ANCA associated vasculitis (A) and IgAV-N (B).

is segmental necrotizing glomerulonephritis. Characteristic findings include inflammatory perfusion of both glomeruli and interstitial tissue, fibrinoid necrosis of glomeruli, glomerular capillary obstruction and crescents. Granulomas are also found in GPA and EGPA. It is worth mentioning again that, because AAV are pauci-immune vasculitides, immunofluorescence is negative, that meaning there is a paucity or absence of glomerular immune deposits. Nevertheless, there are patients who demonstrate atypical histopathological features, such as interstitial nephritis with vasa recta vasculitis. These patients eventually develop the classical lesions of AAV [9, 11, 12] (**Figure 1**).

8. Biomarkers in AAV

Any substance that can be objectively measured and evaluated as an indicator of normal and pathogenic processes or response to an intervention can be used as a biomarker [13].

Inflammatory markers, such as erythrocyte sedimentation rate (ESR) and c-reactive protein (CRP), are non-specific and, although they can be used in the diagnosis of AAV, when evaluated together with clinical and pathological presentation, they are of no value in the differential diagnosis and assessment of disease activity and relapse in diagnosed patients [14].

On the contrary, research on platelet (PLT) counts, which are an acknowledged inflammatory marker, found elevated PLT counts in patients with active disease, compared to patients in remission, and also elevated PLT counts in AAV patients with active disease, compared to AAV patients with infection, thus highlighting their role as an AAV specific marker of disease activity [15].

9. ANCA as biomarkers

Although ANCA are important in the diagnosis of AAV, there are seronegative patients with clinically and pathologically established disease. Furthermore, because diagnosed patients tend to remain ANCA-positive during clinical remission, the use of ANCA as a marker of disease activity and relapse is also limited. Nevertheless, increased values of ANCA in seropositive patients or emergence in seronegative patients, can be evaluated as a marker of disease relapse [14]. Studies have suggested that increase of ANCA titer should not be taken into consideration in terms of changing treatment decisions, but could be used to select patients requiring closer monitoring [14, 16].

10. LAMP-2

Unlike PR3 and MPO, LAMP-2 is also expressed in glomerular endothelial cells, an important site of inflammatory injury [17]. As mentioned before, anti-LAMP-2 antibodies are believed to be formatted through molecular mimicking of bacterial proteins, proposing the implication of this mechanism in the pathogenesis of disease.

One study indicated that anti-LAMP-2 antibodies are present in 80–90% of untreated patients, including PR3-ANCA negative and MPO-ANCA negative patients, while being undetected in healthy controls. Interestingly, anti-LAMP-2antibodies become rapidly undetectable after immunosuppressive therapy, thus suggesting a possible role in the diagnosis and monitoring of AAV patients. However, these findings were not replicated by other investigators, meaning that the use of these antibodies as a biomarker of disease activity is rather inappropriate [10, 14, 17].

11. Plasminogen

The presence of anti-plasminogen antibodies, in about 18–26% of AAV patients, depending on the study, is strongly correlated with glomerular lesion severity, but only weakly correlated with ESR, renal function and renal histopathology [14].

12. Moesin

Moesin, a heparin-binding protein linking actin to the plasma membrane of the cellular cortex, is identified as a possible molecule responsible for the formation of MPO-ANCA, using molecular-mimicking mechanisms, similarly to LAMP-2. Anti-moesin antibodies are found increased in both active AAV disease and remission, but are associated with renal damage, as assessed by correlation to blood urea nitrogen, serum creatinine and proteinuria [14, 18].

13. NET

The contribution of NET in the pathogenesis of AAV is already mentioned. Excessive NET formation is observed in both PR3-ANCA and MPO-ANCA positive patients with active AAV compared to healthy individuals, which is interestingly independent of ANCA titers. Moreover, excessive NET formation is presented in hospitalized AAV patients for disease relapse, but not for infection, suggesting a specificity of NET as a marker of autoimmunity, rather than infection [19].

14. Leucocytes

Regulatory B cells (Bregs) have been investigated as a potential biomarker of AAV. A research group found CD25+ B cells to be increased during disease remission, compared to active disease and healthy controls. Another study revealed CD5+ B cells numerical deficiency in AAV patients, compared to healthy controls. These data, however, are insufficient for the establishment of Bregs as biomarkers in AAV [14, 17].

A study attempted to clarify the role of CD8+ T cells as a biomarker of AAV. The presence of particular gene expression profiles of CD8+ T cells were associated with disease relapse, among patients with the same disease activity, inflammatory markers and treatment. If validated, these data could be used to identify patients in need of customized therapeutic regimens [14, 17, 20].

Regulatory T cells (Tregs) have also been studied by researchers. Decreased number and impaired functionality of Tregs was found in patients with active AAV. Furthermore, the proportion of Tregs was found inversely correlated with relapse and positively associated with time of remission. Based on these data, Tregs could be used as a biomarker of therapeutic and prognostic importance [14, 17].

15. Monocytes

The role of monocytes in the pathogenesis and tissue damage in AAV has already been discussed. Soluble and cell surface markers of monocyte activation are increased in AAV patients, even during disease remission. Furthermore, monocyte-derived macrophages and giant cells within affected tissues and granulomas may be responsible for maintaining autoimmunity. These data suggest that monocytes may account for disease relapse, thus be used as a prognostic biomarker of negative outcome [21].

16. Inflammatory response

- **Complement**: Plasma levels of C3a, C5a, soluble C5b-9 and Bbare found increased in patients with active disease, compared to patients with disease remission and healthy controls [14, 17]. C5a receptor (C5aR) expression is found lower in renal tissue of patients with active disease [17, 22]. Furthermore, plasma levels of Bb, which is indicative of alternative pathway activation, is associated with serum inflammatory markers and the presence of crescents in renal biopsy. Similarly, urinary levels of Bb are positively correlated with serum creatinine levels, indicative of renal function, and negatively correlated with the percentage of normal glomeruli in renal biopsy [14, 17].

- **Monocyte chemotactic protein-1**: Monocyte chemotactic protein-1 (MCP-1), as declared by its name, affects the monocyte/macrophage migration to the tissues. It is also related to the number of circulating monocytes and T cells. Serum MCP-1 is measured significantly higher in patients with AAV, compared to healthy controls. Interestingly, in AAV patients, MCP-1 is found elevated in those with renal involvement, compared to patients without renal involvement. Moreover, serum MCP-1 levels are correlated with serum creatinine levels and proteinuria severity [23].

- **Calprotectin**: Calprotectin is a heterodimer complex of two calcium-binding proteins, expressed on neutrophils, monocytes and early differentiated macrophages [14, 24]. Serum calprotectin is found increased in patients with active AAV and decreased, but not normalized, during remission, thus implicating subclinical disease [24]. Calprotectin levels are, additionally, elevated in patients who discontinued treatment [24] and in patients who relapsed [9, 19], with the elevation predictive of relapse happening during remission [14]. Correlation between calprotectin expression and renal biopsy indicates higher expression of calprotectin in patients with focal lesions and crescents and lower expression in patients with sclerotic findings. Furthermore, neutrophil and monocyte cell surface calprotectin expression is, also, higher in patients with AAV, compared to healthy individuals [24].

- **Neutrophil gelatinase-associated lipocalin**: Neutrophil gelatinase-associated lipocalin (NGAL) is a protein contained in neutrophil granules and, because of its primary secretion, is considered a marker of neutrophil degranulation. Serum levels of NGAL are higher at initial onset and disease relapse of AAV, compared to disease remission, thus suggesting a role in AAV diagnosis and evaluation of activity. Moreover, they are associated with disease severity, ESR, CPR and ANCA titers [25].

- **Angiopoietin-2**: Angiopoietin-2 (Ang-2), an important regulator of endothelial activation, is also positively associated with AAV severity. However, levels of Ang-2 do not decline after successful therapy, thus are not predictive of response to therapy, and, moreover, levels during remission are not predictive of relapse onset [26].

17. Other serum inflammatory proteins

Among many serum inflammatory proteins, such as cytokine, chemokines, soluble receptors, etc., CXCL13 (BCA-1), matrix metalloproteinase-3 (MMP-3) and tissue inhibitor of metalloproteinases-1 (TIMP-1) report the strongest correlation with AAV. Specifically, higher levels of these proteins are found in patients with active disease, compared to healthy individuals, and are also able to distinguish active disease from disease remission. Additionally, lower levels are measured after successful therapy of AAV [14, 27].

18. Urinary biomarkers

A study investigated the role of four urinary proteins [alpha-1 acid glycoprotein (AGP), kidney injury molecule-1 (KIM-1), MCP-1 and NGAL (with the last two being already mentioned above as serum biomarkers)] as biomarkers of active disease. All four proteins were found increased in the urine of patients during active renal disease, compared to remission, with MCP-1 being the most accurate discriminator between the two [23]. MCP-1 levels were also strongly indicative of poor outcome and disease relapse [14, 17, 28].

Another research studied the possible use of urinary soluble CD163 (sCD163), secreted by monocytes and macrophages, as a biomarker in small vessel vasculitis (SVV). Glomeruli of patients with SVV contained remarkably higher levels of CD163 RNA, thus presented increased expression of CD163, than those of patients from disease controls (lupus nephritis, diabetic nephropathy, nephrotic syndrome) [29]. In addition, patients with active SSV had higher levels of urinary sCD163, compared to patients in disease remission [14, 29], disease controls and healthy controls [29].

Urinary excretion of angiogenic factors (VEGF, EGF), cytokines with known pro-inflammatory (IL-6, MCP-1, MIP-1b), anti-inflammatory (IL-2, IL-4, IL-15), and pro-fibrotic activity (TGF-β, IL-6) have been evaluated as biomarkers in renal

Cytokine (pg/mg Ucr)	RPGN n = 38	Controls n = 10	p
IL-2	0.003 ± 0.01	0	0.04
IL-4	0.003 ± 0.006	0.008 ± 0.001	0.04
IL-6	1.2 ± 0.03	0.001 ± 0.001	0.05
IL-8	0.94 ± 2.8	0.04 ± 0.09	0.05
IL-9	0.9 ± 0.0001	0.04 ± 0.09	0.02
IL-15	0.2 ± 0.5	0	0.03
TGF-β1	27.5 ± 79	0.02 ± 0.05	0.04
VEGF	4.3 ± 3.6	0.001 ± 0.0007	<0.0001
MCP-1	2.5 ± 0.001	0.1 ± 0.04	0.01
MIP-1β	1.6 ± 0.001	0.06 ± 0.05	0.02
EGF	0.15 ± 0.3	0.14 ± 0.07	NS

Table 2.
Differences in the urinary excretion between patients with rapidly progressive glomerulonephritis due to vasculitis and controls.

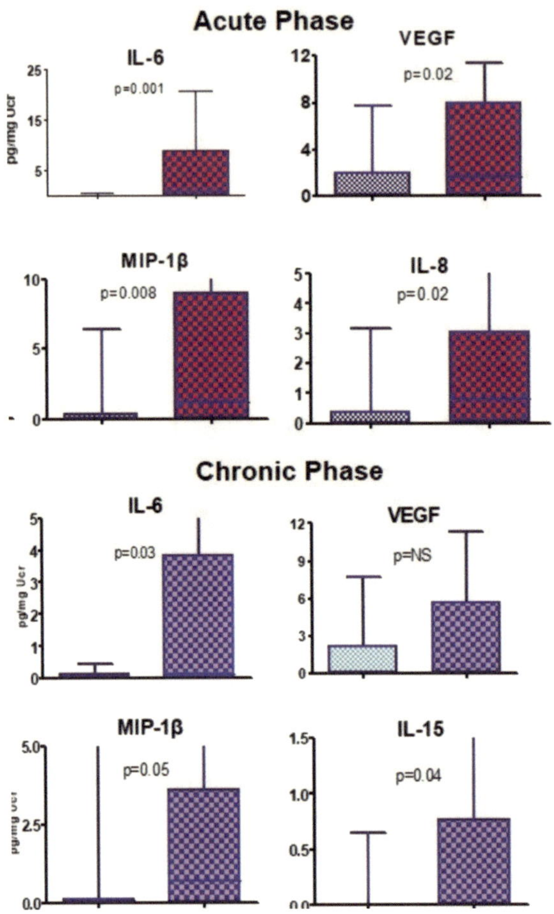

Figure 2.
Impact of cytokines during the acute and chronic phase of vasculitis.

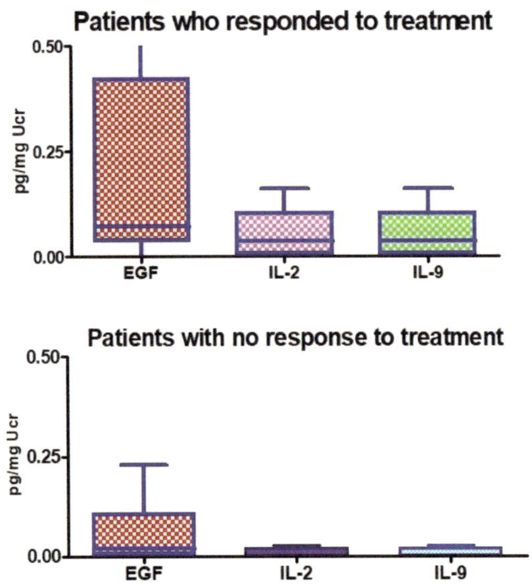

Figure 3.
Favorable influence of cytokines in renal function outcome.

vasculitis. Most of them were significantly increased compared to controls (**Table 2**). Cytokines with possible impact to histologic findings were TGF-β1, IL-15, MCP-1, MIP-1b and EGF. Several factors, such as IL-6, VEGF, MIP-1b and IL-15 could predict worse outcome of renal function, while others, including EGF, IL-2 and IL-9 were correlated with a favorable outcome (**Figures 2** and **3**). The above findings suggested that these factors may act synergistically or competitively during the progression of the disease [30, 31].

19. IgA vasculitis-nephritis

Immunoglobulin A vasculitis-nephritis (IgAV-N), formerly known as Henoch-Schonlein purpura nephritis (HSPN) is the most common vasculitis in childhood, with an annual incidence of 13–20/100,000 children under 17 years of age, but also affects adults and elderly patients with increasing incidence. IgAV is a small vessel vasculitis, usually presents by palpable purpura on the lower legs, arthritis, abdominal pain, and nephritis, while less frequent are manifestations from pulmonary involvement, such as alveolar hemorrhage and neurologic involvement [32–34].

Diagnosis of the IgAV-N is mainly based on the criteria defined by The European League Against Rheumatism (EULAR), Paediatric Rheumatology International Trials Organization (PRINTO) and Paediatric Rheumatology European Society (PRES) (EULAR/PRI NTO/PRES) [35, 36].

Among children with IgAV a proportion of 20–60% will show renal complications, most of them occur at disease onset. Manifestations of renal involvement cover a wide spectrum of symptoms ranging from urinary abnormalities, such as hematuria or/and proteinuria, to rapidly progressive glomerulonephritis and acute kidney disease. Although disease is considered as mild and self-limited, a considerable proportion reaching to 15% will develop chronic kidney disease. The presence of nephritic syndrome, impaired renal function at presentation, increased levels of proteinuria, severe histology and no response to treatment are considered as parameters predicting adverse outcome of renal function [32, 34].

20. Renal pathology

Histology of IgAV-N is characterized by mesangial hypercellularity and mesangial deposition of IgA and C3, with or without IgG. Fibrinoid necrosis and crescents are a common finding, while the presence of segmental or global sclerosis, endocapillary hyperplasia, severity of tubulointerstital fibrosis and inflammatory infiltration may vary between cases (**Figure 1**) [35, 36].

Several classification systems have attempted to organize histological findings and evaluate their significance. The classification proposed by the International Study of Kidney Disease in Children (ISKDC), mainly based on the presence and extent of crescents, is widely used, although lately there have been attempts to apply Oxford classification system in IgAV-N, in the same way as this is used for IgAN classification [35].

According to ISKDC classification, optical microscopy findings are categorized into six histological grades. Grades I-V are based on the extension of crescents, grade VI describes a membranoproliferative type glomerulonephritis. The system was designed to estimate vasculitic lesions and inflammation, therefore it took into account the state of glomeruli only and not tubulointerstitial lesions. This seems to be the main disadvantage of the system, as presence and percentage of crescent formation merely reflect active inflammation, and their predictive value has been doubted in recent studies, which showed that patients on higher grades may experience spontaneous remission, while those with low grade histologic lesions may develop chronic renal failure [37–40].

The Oxford classification system, available since 2009, has been designed to estimate histology in IgAN, and it was based initially on four morphologic features: mesangial hypercellularity (M), endocapillary proliferation (E), segmental glomerulosclerosis (S) and tubular atrophy/interstitial fibrosis (T), which formed the MEST score [41–43]. More recently, the system was revised to MEST-C score, including the present of crescents, as crescent score (C) [44]. Although patients with IgAV-N were not included in the validation cohort, and therefore, the classification system cannot officially be recommend for patients with this condition, there have been few recent attempts to apply Oxford classification in IgAV-N. The presence of endocapillary proliferation and tubulointerstitial fibrosis were the main histologic findings associated with worse outcome of renal function [44–46].

Renal biopsy is essential for diagnosing IgAV-N, probably guide treatment and predict outcome, but, the procedure cannot be used repeatedly during follow up of the patients. The use of biomarkers is again mandatory to estimate disease outcome. IgAV-N share the same pathogenic pathway with IgAN, mediated by aberrant O-linked glycosylation of IgA1 hinge region, they are considered similar diseases that share common pathophysiologic mechanisms. Based on this fact, researchers tried to evaluate the utility of IgAN biomarkers in the assessment of the clinical course of IgAV-N. It was thus found that several of them could be used in IgAV-N patients as well [47, 48].

21. Biomarkers in IgAV-N

21.1 Serum and urine immunoglobins and immune complexes

Since IgA deposition in various tissues is an important parameter of the disease pathophysiology, several studies have tried to examine immunoglobin production in IgAV patients. It has been found that IgA and IgE serum concentrations are higher in individuals with IgAV compared to normal controls, although it has not been proven that they can be useful in distinguishing patients with and without nephritis [47]. Moreover, serum Gd-IgA1 and IgA-IgG complexes, as well as urine IgA and IgA-IgG complexes are potential biomarkers for IgAV-N. More specifically, elevated levels of Gd-IgA1 in the blood of IgAV patients have been correlated with the presence of nephritis [47]. It has been proposed that recognition of the under galactosylated IgA1 hinge region by IgA or IgG antibodies induces the production of circulating immune complexes [47, 48]. Indeed, high concentrations of IgA-IgG complexes have been found in the serum of all IgAV-N patients, while in urine, the levels of these complexes are increased only in patients who have developed nephritis [47, 48]. It seems though that deterioration of renal function is not associated with the serum levels of Gd-IgA1 and IgA-IgG complexes. Recently, a French multicenter prospective study showed that urinary IgA concentration can be used as an additional index in order to improve patient risk stratification for poor outcome at disease onset. This is an important finding, since only a small percentage of IgAV patients finally develop severe deterioration of renal function and can benefit from intensive care, monitoring and follow-up and for the time IgAV outcome assessment is based on conventional clinical factors [48].

22. Cluster of differentiation (CD) antigens

Concerning CD antigens that could be used as biomarkers, CD89 has been found to be useful in the assessment of IgAV. CD89 is the human myeloid specific IgA Fc receptor. It is expressed on neutrophils, eosinophils, monocytes/macrophages, dendritic cells and Kupffer cells [49, 50]. In IgAN patients, cleavage of the CD89 extracellular domain and release of IgA-soluble CD89 (IgA-sCD89) complexes is caused by the binding of IgA to CD89. Therefore, high levels of circulating IgA-sCD89 complexes are observed in these patients. The complexes are trapped in the mesangium by the transferin receptor. Their deposition, as well as mesangial activation, is facilitated by transglutaminase 2 (TG2) [48, 51]. IgAV patients demonstrate decreased expression of CD89 at their monocyte and granulocyte cell surface. This finding is combined with increased blood concentration of IgA-sCD89 complexes. Urinary levels of these complexes are more elevated in individuals who develop nephritis [47, 48]. Furthermore, according to the findings of a 2016 multicenter study, urinary CD89 and TG2 concentrations are significantly lower in patients with active IgA vasculitis with nephritis (IgAV-N) compared to individuals whose disease has gone into complete or partial remission. More specifically, urinary CD89 and TG2 levels were found to be positively correlated with each other and negatively correlated with the level of proteinuria. It has been proposed that this decrease is consistent with the reduction in CD89 and TG2 urinary excretion as a result of the mononuclear-cell mediated inflammatory reaction that is induced by IgA-sCD89 deposition in the kidney. During this active phase, large multimolecular complexes containing CD89, TG2, CD71 and IgA1 are stabilized on the mesangial cell surface, thus causing CD89 and TG2 molecules to remain in the renal tissue. Interestingly, there seems to be a stronger negative correlation between proteinuria and urinary CD89 levels in comparison to TG2 levels, thus suggesting that CD89 might decrease earlier in the urine of patients with IgAV-N [51].

CD62L (L-selectin) and CD11b are also found to be upregulated in IgAN patients and are considered to be involved in IgAV pathogenesis. CD62L, is an adhesion molecule observed on the neutrophil surface that mediates the initial adhesion of neutrophils to the endothelium and could consequently be important in the early development of IgAV. CD11b is a predominant β2 integrin, also expressed on neutrophils. High CD11b and IgA levels possibly promote vascular damage through induction of antibody-dependent cellular toxicity (ADCC) [52].

23. Cytokines and other inflammatory factors

Regarding pro-inflammatory cytokines, IgAV patients with or without nephritis present high serum concentrations of IL-1b, IL-6 and IL-8 compared with normal controls, with the increase in IL-6 and IL-8 levels being very significant in individuals with renal involvement. Urine IL-6, IL-8 and IL-10 concentrations appear to be more elevated in IgAV-N patients, in the same way as in patients with IgAN [53, 54]. These cytokines possibly play a role in mesangial cell activation, proliferation, crescent formation and glomerulosclerosis. Additionally, increase in IL-6 blood concentration seems to be an index of the acute phase of IgAV [47, 48]. Tumor necrosis factor (TNF) blood levels, that have also been associated with the development of interstitial fibrosis and tubular atrophy regardless of renal function, are higher in IgAV patients who present with nephritis [47]. Furthermore, several other inflammatory parameters, including C-reactive protein (CRP), Serum Amyloid A (SAA) and Neutrophil-Lymphocyte ratio (NLR), also seem to be upregulated in IgAV patients in comparison to healthy individuals [55]. Of all these inflammatory indexes, NLR seems to present the strongest diagnostic value concerning the development of extracutaneal manifestations in adult IgAV (gastrointestinal and/or renal). The severity of the systemic involvement has been found to be associated with high NLR before treatment [56]. There is also a possible connection between high SAA levels also has a possible connection with the presence of gastrointestinal manifestations [52].

24. Neutrophil gelatinase-associated lipocalin (NGAL)

NGAL protein, a member of the lipocalin superfamily initially found in activated neutrophils, is produced in various cell types including renal tubules. It is a factor promoting kidney cellular proliferation and differentiation that is significantly upregulated in response to epithelial injury, thus serving as an index of kidney damage [47, 57]. It can possibly predict the appearance of acute renal impairment and the acute deterioration of unstable nephropathies. Furthermore, it may also be implicated in the pathophysiology of some chronic kidney disease (CKD) conditions, such as polycystic kidney disease and glomerulonephritis, while its levels are directly associated with the degree of renal damage [25]. In IgAV, NGAL concentrations seem to be high in both patients with and without nephritis, while its levels in urine, found more elevated in patients with nephritis, are useful in distinguishing them from individuals without kidney impairment [47, 48].

25. Soluble transferin receptor (sTfR)

sTfR consists of a single polypeptide chain and has been found to be upregulated in IgAV-N and IgAN patients, perhaps as a result of IgA1 polymer-mediated induction. Its overexpression is thought to be associated with the disease severity. Normally, it cannot cross the glomerular membrane because of its molecular size. However, when non-selective glomerular proteinuria is present, it is possible that the molecule can passively cross the membrane and then be detected in the urine. Interestingly, it has been found that in IgAV-N and IgAN patients the sTfR/creatinine ratio is higher than the ratio measured in healthy individuals or patients with other glomerulopathies. Therefore, it can possibly be used as a non-invasive tool to distinguish those two diseases from other pathologies that cause proteinuria. It has also been proposed that sTfR can additionally be further evaluated as a potential prognostic and activity marker for IgAV-N and IgAN [58].

Author details

Polyvios Arseniou[1], Stamatia Stai[1] and Maria Stangou[1,2]*

1 School of Medicine, Aristotle University of Thessaloniki, Greece

2 Department of Nephrology, Hippokration Hospital, Aristotle University of Thessaloniki, Greece

*Address all correspondence to: mstangou@auth.gr

References

[1] Zhang J, Defelice AF, Hanig JP, Colatsky T. Biomarkers of endothelial cell activation serve as potential surrogate markers for drug-induced vascular injury. Toxicologic Pathology. 2010;**38**(6):856-871

[2] Mariani LH, Kretzler M. Pro: 'The usefulness of biomarkers in glomerular diseases'. The problem: Moving from syndrome to mechanism—Individual patient variability in disease presentation, course and response to therapy. Nephrology, Dialysis, Transplantation. 2015;**30**(6):892-898

[3] Piéroni L, Cristol JP. Urinary biomarkers of kidney dysfunction. Annales de biologie clinique (Paris). 2015;**73**(2):151-157

[4] Zhang J, Hanig JP, De Felice AF. Biomarkers of endothelial cell activation: Candidate markers for drug-induced vasculitis in patients or drug-induced vascular injury in animals. Vascular Pharmacology. 2012;**56**(1-2):14-25

[5] Biasucci LM, Cardillo MT. Biomarkers of inflammation and endothelial function: The holy grail of experimental and clinical medicine? Vascular Pharmacology. 2012;**56**(1-2):26-28

[6] Jarrot P, Kaplanski G. Pathogenesis of ANCA-associated vasculitis: An update. Autoimmunity Reviews. 2016;**15**(7):704-713

[7] Kallenberg C. Anti-neutrophil cytoplasmic antibody (ANCA)-associated vasculitis: Where to go? Clinical and Experimental Immunology. 2011;**164**:1-3

[8] Pendergraft W, Nachman P. Recent pathogenetic advances in ANCA-associated vasculitis. La Presse Médicale. 2015;**44**(6):e223-e229

[9] Rowaiye O, Kusztal M, Klinger M. The kidneys and ANCA-associated vasculitis: From pathogenesis to diagnosis. Clinical Kidney Journal. 2015;**8**(3):343-350

[10] Salama A, Pusey C. Shining a LAMP on pauci-immune focal segmental glomerulonephritis. Kidney International. 2009;**76**(1):15-17

[11] Zonozi R, Niles J, Cortazar F. Renal involvement in antineutrophil cytoplasmic antibody-associated vasculitis. Rheumatic Disease Clinics of North America. 2018;**44**(4):525-543

[12] Stangou M. Systemic vasculitides with renal involvment. In: Internal Medicine. 5th ed. Thessaloniki, Greece: University Studio Press; 2017. pp. 447-449

[13] Brogan P, Eleftheriou D. Vasculitis update: Pathogenesis and biomarkers. Pediatric Nephrology. 2017;**33**(2):187-198

[14] Draibe J, Fulladosa X, Cruzado J, Torras J, Salama A. Current and novel biomarkers in anti-neutrophil cytoplasm-associated vasculitis. Clinical Kidney Journal. 2016;**9**(4):547-551

[15] Willeke P, Kümpers P, Schlüter B, Limani A, Becker H, Schotte H. Platelet counts as a biomarker in ANCA-associated vasculitis. Scandinavian Journal of Rheumatology. 2015;**44**(4):302-308. DOI: 10.3109/03009742.2015.1006247

[16] Tomasson G, Grayson P, Mahr A, LaValley M, Merkel P. Value of ANCA measurements during remission to predict a relapse of ANCA-associated vasculitis—A meta-analysis. Rheumatology. 2011;**51**(1):100-109. DOI: 10.1093/rheumatology/ker280

[17] Lally L, Spiera R. Biomarkers in ANCA-associated vasculitis. Current

Rheumatology Reports. 2013;**15**(10):363. DOI: 10.1007/s11926-013-0363-x

[18] Suzuki K, Suzuki K, Nagao T, Nakayama T. Proposal of anti-moesin as a novel biomarker for ANCA-associated vasculitis. Clinical and Experimental Nephrology. 2013;**17**(5):638-641. DOI: 10.1007/s10157-013-0861-1

[19] Kraaij T, Kamerling S, van Dam L, Bakker J, Bajema I, Page T, et al. Excessive neutrophil extracellular trap formation in ANCA-associated vasculitis is independent of ANCA. Kidney International. 2018;**94**(1):139-149. DOI: 10.1016/j.kint.2018.01.013

[20] Chen A, Lee K, Guan T, He J, Schlondorff D. Role of CD8⁺ T cells in crescentic glomerulonephritis. Nephrology, Dialysis, Transplantation. 16 Mar 2019. pii: gfz043. DOI: 10.1093/ndt/gfz043

[21] Brunini F, Page T, Gallieni M, Pusey C. The role of monocytes in ANCA-associated vasculitides. Autoimmunity Reviews. 2016;**15**(11):1046-1053. DOI: 10.1016/j.autrev.2016.07.031

[22] Dick J, Gan P, Ford S, Odobasic D, Alikhan M, Loosen S, et al. C5a receptor 1 promotes autoimmunity, neutrophil dysfunction and injury in experimental anti-myeloperoxidase glomerulonephritis. Kidney International. 2018;**93**(3):615-625

[23] Liu S, Li N, Zhu Q, Zhu B, Wu T, Wang G, et al. Increased serum MCP-1 levels in systemic vasculitis patients with renal involvement. Journal of Interferon and Cytokine Research. 2018;**38**(9):406-412

[24] Pepper R, Hamour S, Chavele K, Todd S, Rasmussen N, Flint S, et al. Leukocyte and serum S100A8/S100A9 expression reflects disease activity in ANCA-associated vasculitis and glomerulonephritis. Kidney International. 2013, 2013;**83**(6):1150-1158

[25] Chen M, Wang F, Zhao M. Circulating neutrophil gelatinase-associated lipocalin: A useful biomarker for assessing disease activity of ANCA-associated vasculitis. Rheumatology. 2009;**48**(4):355-358

[26] Monach P, Kümpers P, Lukasz A, Tomasson G, Specks U, Stone J, et al. Circulating angiopoietin-2 as a biomarker in ANCA-associated vasculitis. PLoS ONE. 2012;**7**(1):e30197. DOI: 10.1371/journal.pone.0030197

[27] Monach P, Warner R, Tomasson G, Specks U, Stone J, Ding L, et al. Serum proteins reflecting inflammation, injury and repair as biomarkers of disease activity in ANCA-associated vasculitis. Annals of the Rheumatic Diseases. 2013;**72**(8):1342-1350

[28] Lieberthal J, Cuthbertson D, Carette S, Hoffman G, Khalidi N, Koening C, et al. Urinary biomarkers in relapsing antineutrophil cytoplasmic antibody-associated vasculitis. The Journal of Rheumatology. 2013;**40**(5):674-683. DOI: 10.3899/jrheum.120879

[29] O'Reilly V, Wong L, Kennedy C, Elliot L, O'Meachair S, Coughlan A, et al. Urinary soluble CD163 in active renal vasculitis. Journal of the American Society of Nephrology. 2016;**27**(9):2906-2916

[30] Stangou M, Papagianni A, Bantis C, Liakou H, Pliakos K, Giamalis P, et al. Detection of multiple cytokines in the urine of patients with focal necrotising glomerulonephritis may predict short and long term outcome of renal function. Cytokine. 2012;**57**(1):120-126

[31] Stangou M, Bantis C, Skoularopoulou M, Korelidou L, Kouloukouriotou D, Scina M, et al. Th1, Th2 and Treg/T17 cytokines in two types of proliferative glomerulonephritis. Indian Journal Nephrology. 2016;**26**(3):159-166

[32] Nicoara O, Twombley K. Immunoglobulin A nephropathy and immunoglobulin A vasculitis. Pediatric Clinics of North America. 2019;**66**(1):101-110

[33] Heineke MH, Ballering AV, Jamin A, Ben Mkaddem S, Monteiro RC, Van Egmond M. New insights in the pathogenesis of immunoglobulin A vasculitis (Henoch-Schönleinpurpura). Autoimmunity Reviews. 2017;**16**(12):1246-1253

[34] Hetland LE, Susrud KS, Lindahl KH, Bygum A. Henoch-SchönleinPurpura: A literature review. Acta Dermato-Venereologica. 2017;**97**(10):1160-1166

[35] Ozen S, Pistorio A, Lusan SM, Bakkaloglu A, Herlin T, Brik R, et al. EULAR/PRINTO/PRES criteria for Henoch-Schonleinpurpura, childhood polyarteritisnodosa, childhood Wegener granulomatosis and childhood Takayasu arteritis: Ankara 2008. Part I: Overall methodology and clinical characterisation. Annals of the Rheumatic Diseases. 2010;**69**:790-797

[36] Jelusic M, Sestan M, Cimaz R, Ozen S. Different histological classifications for Henoch-Schönleinpurpura nephritis: Which one should be used? Pediatric Rheumatology Online Journal. 2019;**17**(1):10

[37] Mao S, Xuan X, Sha Y, Zhao S, Zhu C, Zhang A, et al. Clinico-pathological association of Henoch-Schoenleinpurpuranephritis and IgA nephropathy in children. International Journal of Clinical and Experimental Pathology. 2015;**8**(3):2334-2342

[38] Ronkainen J, Nuutinen M, Koskimies O. The adult kidney 24 years after childhood Henoch-Schonleinpurpura: A retrospective cohort study. Lancet. 2002;**360**:666-670

[39] Coppo R, Andrulli S, Amore A, Gianoglio B, Conti G, Peruzzi L, et al. Predictors of outcome in Henoch-Schönlein nephritis in children and adults. American Journal of Kidney Diseases. 2006;**47**:993-1003

[40] Soylemezoglu O, Ozkaya O, Ozen S, Bakkaloglu A, Dusunsel R, Peru H, et al. Henoch-Schönlein nephritis: A nationwide study. Nephron. Clinical Practice. 2009;**112**:199-204

[41] Roberts ISD, Cook HT, Troyanov S, Alpers CE, Amore A, Barratt J, et al. The Oxford classification of IgA nephropathy: Pathology definitions, correlations, and reproducibility. Kidney International. 2009;**76**:546-556

[42] Cattran DC, Coppo R, Cook HT, Feehally J, Roberts ISD, Troyanov S, et al. The Oxford classification of IgA nephropathy: Rationale, clinicopathological correlations, and classification. Kidney International. 2009;**76**:534-545

[43] Trimarchi H, Barratt J, Cattran DC, Cook HT, Coppo R, Haas M, et al. Oxford classification of IgA nephropathy 2016: An update from the IgA. Kidney International. 2017;**91**(5):1014-1021

[44] Inagaki K, Kaihan AB, Hachiya A, Ozeki T, Ando M, Kato S, et al. Clinical impact of endocapillary proliferation according to the Oxford classification among adults with Henoch-Schönleinpurpura nephritis: A multicenter retrospective cohort study. BMC Nephrology. 2018;**19**(1):208. DOI: 10.1186/s12882-018-1009-z

[45] Kim CH, Lim BJ, Bae YS, Kwon YE, Kim YL, Nam KH, et al. Using the Oxford classification of IgA nephropathy to predict long-term outcomes of Henoch-Schönlein purpura nephritis in adults. Modern Pathology. 2014;**27**(7):972-982

[46] Nasri H. Oxford classification of IgA nephropathy is applicable

to predict long-term outcomes of Henoch-Schönlein purpura nephritis. Iranian Journal of Allergy, Asthma, and Immunology. 2014;**13**(6):456-458

[47] Pillebout E, Jamin A, Ayari H, Housset P, Pierre M, Sauvaget V, et al. Biomarkers of IgA vasculitis nephritis in children. PLoS ONE. 2017;**12**(11):e0188718. DOI: 10.1371/journal.pone.0188718. eCollection 2017

[48] Berthelot L, Jamin A, Viglietti D, Chemouny JM, Ayari H, Pierre M, et al. Value of biomarkers for predicting immunoglobulin A vasculitis nephritis outcome in an adult prospective cohort. Nephrology, Dialysis, Transplantation. 2018;**33**(9):1579-1590

[49] van de Winkel JG. Fc receptors: Role in biology and antibody therapy. Immunology Letters. 2010;**128**(1):4-5

[50] Monteiro RC, Van De Winkel JG. IgA Fc receptors. Annual Review of Immunology. 2003;**21**:177-204

[51] Moresco RN, Speeckaert MM, Zmonarski SC, Krajewska M, Komuda-Leszek E, Perkowska-Ptasinska A, et al. Urinary myeloid IgA Fc alpha receptor (CD89) and transglutaminase-2 as new biomarkers for active IgA nephropathy and Henoch-Schönleinpurpura nephritis. BBA Clinical. 2016;**5**:79-84

[52] Kuret T, Lakota K, Žigon P, Ogrič M, Sodin-Šemrl S, Čučnik S, et al. Insight into inflammatory cell and cytokine profiles in adult IgA vasculitis. Clin Rheumatology. 2019;**38**(2):331-338

[53] Stangou M, Papagianni A, Bantis C, Moisiadis D, Kasimatis S, Spartalis M, et al. Up-regulation of urinary markers predict outcome in IgA nephropathy but their predictive value is influenced by treatment with steroids and azathioprine. Clinical Nephrology. 2013;**80**(3):203-210

[54] Stangou M, Alexopoulos E, Papagianni A, Pantzaki A, Bantis C, Dovas S, et al. Urinary levels of epidermal growth factor, interleukin-6 and monocyte chemoattractant protein-1 may act as predictor markers of renal function outcome in immunoglobulin A nephropathy. Nephrology (Carlton). 2009;**14**(6):613-620

[55] Purevdorj N, Mu Y, Gu Y, Zheng F, Wang R, Yu J, et al. Clinical significance of the serum biomarker index detection in children with Henoch-Schonleinpurpura. Clinical Biochemistry. 2018;**52**:167-170

[56] Nagy GR, Kemény L, Bata-Csörgő Z. Neutrophil-to-lymphocyte ratio: A biomarker for predicting systemic involvement in adult IgA vasculitis patients. Journal of the European Academy of Dermatology and Venereology. 2017;**31**(6):1033-1037

[57] Bolignano D, Donato V, Coppolino G, Campo S, Buemi A, Lacquaniti A, et al. Neutrophil gelatinase-associated lipocalin (NGAL) as a marker of kidneydamage. American Journal of Kidney Diseases. 2008;**52**(3):595-605

[58] Delanghe SE, Speeckaert MM, Segers H, Desmet K, VandeWalle J, Laecke SV, et al. Soluble transferrin receptor in urine, a new biomarker for IgA nephropathy and Henoch-Schönleinpurpura nephritis. Clinical Biochemistry. 2013;**46**(7-8):591-597

Section 2

Glomerulonephritis in Childhood

Chapter 3

Childhood Idiopathic Nephrotic Syndrome as a Podocytopathy

Samuel N. Uwaezuoke

Abstract

Idiopathic nephrotic syndrome is the commonest manifestation of glomerular disease in children. The syndrome is characterized by massive proteinuria, hypoalbuminemia, generalized edema, and hyperlipidemia. Although genetic or congenital forms are now well recognized, nephrotic syndrome is largely acquired. The latter form can be idiopathic or primary (the causes are unknown) and secondary (the causes are known renal or non-renal diseases). Idiopathic nephrotic syndrome consists of the following glomerulonephritides: minimal change nephropathy (MCN), focal segmental glomerulosclerosis (FSGS), membranoproliferative glomerulonephritis (MPGN), mesangial proliferative glomerulonephritis (MesPGN), and membranous nephritis (MN). The etiopathogenesis of nephrotic syndrome has evolved through several hypotheses ranging from immune dysregulation theory and increased glomerular permeability theory to the current concept of podocytopathy. Podocyte injury is now thought to be the basic pathology in the syndrome. The book chapter aims to highlight the mechanisms underlying the pathogenesis of nephrotic syndrome as a podocytopathy.

Keywords: idiopathic nephrotic syndrome, glomerular disease, glomerulonephritides, podocyte injury

1. Introduction

Nephrotic syndrome is the commonest manifestation of glomerular disease which is characterized by massive proteinuria, hypoalbuminemia, generalized edema, and hyperlipidemia [1]. In children, primary or idiopathic nephrotic syndrome (INS) may be caused by any of these glomerulonephritides: minimal change nephropathy (MCN), focal segmental glomerulosclerosis (FSGS), membranoproliferative glomerulonephritis (MPGN), mesangial proliferative glomerulonephritis (MesPGN), and membranous nephropathy (MN). MCN appears to be the most common histopathologic type, followed by FSGS and MPGN in that order [2–4]. However, recent reports from different parts of the world suggest a change in the pattern of the predominant histopathologic types in childhood INS. For instance, there has been a rise in the prevalence rates of FSGS documented among children in the West African subregion [5–7]. This trend also applies to MPGN [8], a histological subtype hitherto thought to be more common in adult patients.

In the pathogenesis of INS, there is now a paradigm shift from the concept of an immune-dysregulated disease of the glomerular basement membrane to that of a podocytopathy [9, 10]. In fact, it is now assumed that podocyte abnormalities account for all forms of nephrotic syndrome. Basically, the podocyte is involved in maintaining the structural integrity of the glomerular filtration barrier. Thus, podocyte injury and loss result in significant proteinuria as well as progressive glomerulosclerosis [11]. Podocytopathy can occur in immunologic and non-immunologic diseases of the kidney. Acquired podocytopathies such as MCN and FSGS are considered to have immunologic basis [12]. Interestingly, immunosuppressive therapy has been noted to directly affect the podocyte through the regulation of interleukin-4 (IL-4) and interleukin-13 (IL-13) and several signaling pathways involved with the stabilization of the actin cytoskeleton and the distribution of the slit diaphragm components [11]. This book chapter aims to discuss the mechanisms underpinning the pathogenesis of childhood INS as a podocytopathy.

2. The molecular structure and function of the podocyte

The glomerular filtration barrier is essentially a trilaminate structure which consists of the podocyte on the outer surface, the glomerular basement membrane (GBM) in the middle, and the fenestrated endothelium on the inner surface (**Figure 1**). The podocyte (also known as the visceral glomerular epithelial cell) constitutes the last barrier to protein loss, given its unique structure and location as a terminally differentiated cell which lines the outer surface of the GBM. Each podocyte comprises the foot processes which are separated by a filtration slit (or the slit diaphragm). The foot process comprises components such as actin, myosin-II, α-actinin-4, talin, and vinculin which all constitute a contractile structure [13]. The filament bundles which make up actin are disposed together as arches between contiguous podocyte foot processes [14] and are connected to the GBM at specific points through an adhesion molecule (α-3β-1 integrin complex) [15, 16]. Similarly, the linkage of the podocyte foot processes to the GBM is made possible through both α-3β-1 integrin and dystroglycans [17]. Adjacent foot processes are linked by the slit diaphragm, which forms the main size-selective filter barrier in the glomerular architecture [18, 19]. The filtration slit is composed of multiple protein molecules such as nephrin, P-cadherin, CD2AP, ZO-1, FAT, podocin, and possibly

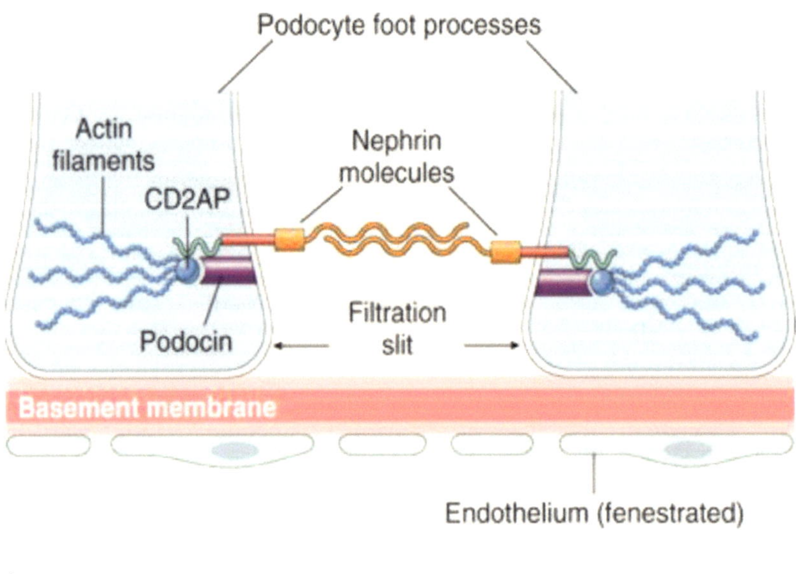

Figure 1.
Schematic representation of the molecular structure of the glomerular filtration barrier (Courtesy: Flickr photos).

Neph1 [20–22]. In addition, synaptopodin is closely related to the actin filaments located within the podocyte foot processes [23] and interacts with the tight junction protein, MAGI-1, in the same way as α-actinin-4 MAGI-1 being expressed in podocytes as well [24]. The functional integrity of the podocytes depends on the actin cytoskeleton. This is critical in preserving the intact glomerular filtration barrier, as a healthy podocyte is essential for the maintenance of this barrier.

2.1 The molecular mechanisms in podocytopathy

Among the fundamental biologic events in INS, a molecular disruption of the filtration slit or GBM results in proteinuria, while rearrangement of podocyte cytoskeleton accounts for foot process effacement. In fact, the basic role played by the podocyte actin cytoskeleton (the skeletal structure of the foot processes) in the pathogenesis of INS is predicated on the disruption of actin-related proteins with the GBM, resulting in effacement of the podocyte foot processes [25]. Still at the molecular level, focal adhesion kinase (FAK) plays an essential role in this foot process effacement, usually observed in podocytopathies [26]. Furthermore, alterations in podocyte proteins such as nephrin and Neph1 (nephrin homologue), CD2-associated protein (CD2AP), and podocin all contribute to the pathogenesis of INS as podocytopathies [27–29]. Nephrin represents an essential constituent of the slit diaphragm and also serves as an efficient mobilizer of other proteins such as podocin and CD2AP (**Figure 1**) [30]. It has been proposed that a vital interaction exists between the actin cytoskeleton and the molecules that make up the filtration slit such as podocin, nephrin, and CD2AP [31, 32]. Thus, nephrotic-range proteinuria occurs as a result of structural disruptions in the podocytes which present as foot process effacement, as well as changes in the actin cytoskeleton and molecular alteration of the filtration slit [33]. Again, the component molecules of the actin cytoskeleton include actin, α-actinin, and synaptopodin [34, 35]. Interestingly, the upregulation of α-actinin results in the reorganization of the cytoskeleton in some nephrotic syndromes [36], while the expression of synaptopodin is generally preserved in MCN, but diminished in FSGS [37]. Podocalyxin is a molecule presumed to mediate the stability of the foot processes [38] and has also been found to be raised in nephrotic syndromes [39]. Finally, the fundamental role of adhesion molecules such as integrins and focal adhesion proteins has been shown in genetically based animal experiments which end up in nephrotic syndrome [40, 41]. Specifically, α3β1 (the main integrin heterodimer in the podocyte), when destroyed in the podocytes of experimental mice, gave rise to nephrotic-range proteinuria and foot process effacement. In addition, αvβ3 integrin (also expressed in podocytes) can be activated by uroplasminogen type I activator receptor (uPAR) (in podocytes) [42] or its soluble form, suPAR (from the circulation) [43]. Its activation notably leads to foot process effacement through the rearrangement of the podocyte actin cytoskeleton: a characteristic event in podocytopathy [44].

3. Treatment targets in the podocytopathy model

Interventions targeting molecular pathways which regulate the actin cytoskeleton can potentially play an important role in the treatment of proteinuric kidney diseases, such as nephrotic syndrome. There are three major molecular frameworks which modulate the actin cytoskeleton and prevent podocyte detachment from GBM, namely, Rho-GTPases, cell-matrix adhesion proteins, and endocytic proteins. For instance, the podocyte-expressed RhoA, Rac1, and Cdc42 regulate signal transduction pathways which affect many aspects of cell behavior, including alterations in the actin cytoskeleton [45, 46]. The regulatory ability of these protein molecules on the actin cytoskeleton points to their fundamental role in the pathogenesis of nephrotic syndrome and as possible treatment targets [25]. For instance, the inhibition of RhoA and Rac1 could potentially reduce proteinuria and optimize renal function and ameliorate glomerulopathy [47–50], given that elevated RhoA activity has been noted to induce foot process effacement and subsequent proteinuria [51].

Furthermore, blocking αvβ3 integrin with an anti-β3 antibody or cilengitide (the small molecule inhibitor) was noted to have ameliorated uPAR-induced proteinuria, underscoring the importance of this integrin as another potential therapeutic target [42, 43]. Also, targeted pharmacologic inhibition of integrin α2β1 in murine models also reduced proteinuria [52], while inhibition of major focal adhesion proteins, such as FAK and Crk1/Crk2, reduced both podocyte foot process effacement and proteinuria [26, 53]. In addition, one important therapeutic target in proteinuria is the regulating activation of integrin β1 via abatacept (CTLA-4-Ig) or integrin αv inhibitor, cilengitide, or integrin α2β1 [42, 43, 52, 54].

The link between transient receptor potential cation channels (TRPCs) and the actin cytoskeleton has also been well reported [25]. TRPCs are nonselective cationic channels with affinity for calcium ions, which contribute significantly in the pathogenesis of renal and cardiovascular diseases [55]. In podocytes, many

Potential pharmacologic agents	Treatment targets in podocytopathy	Indications	Efficacy	Side effects
Cyclosporine A† (a major calcineurin inhibitor. Another example is FK 506)	Downregulation of synaptopodin	Clinical use in SRNS and in renal transplantation	Induces remission in SRNS	Major side effects in humans: tremors, hypertension, nephrotoxicity, hirsutism, and gum hypertrophy
Inhibitors of small Rho-GTPases‡	Small Rho-GTPases (Rho A, Rac 1)	Still under trial (nephrotic syndrome)	–	–
Cilengitide/anti-β3 antibody*	Blockage of αvβ3 integrin	Still under trial (nephrotic syndrome) Clinical use in glioblastoma	–	–
Abatacept	Modulating activation of integrin β1	Still under trial/ clinical use in FSGS	–	–
Inhibitors of TRPC 5**	TRPC 5	Still under trial	–	–
Bis-T-23	Dynamin oligomerization and actin polymerization	Still under trial 1 (proteinuric kidney diseases, CKD)	–	–

†Protects synaptopodin from cathepsin L-mediated degradation (stabilizes actin cytoskeleton).
‡Potentially ameliorates proteinuria.
**Reduces uroplasminogen type 1 activator receptor-induced proteinuria/also inhibits angiogenesis.*
***Protects against liposaccharide-induced proteinuria and foot process effacement (adapted from Ref. [68]).*
SRNS, steroid-resistant nephrotic syndrome; CKD, chronic kidney disease; FK 506, nitrogen mustard and tacrolimus; FSGS, focal segmental glomerulosclerosis; TRPC, transient receptor potential cation channel

Table 1.
Summary of current and future treatment targets and the potential drugs for idiopathic nephrotic syndrome.

TRPCs are reportedly expressed, namely, TRPC1, TRPC3, TRPC4, TRPC5, and TRPC6 [56–60]. A striking therapeutic application is the ability of TRPC5 inhibitor (ML204) to protect against lipopolysaccharide (LPS)-induced proteinuria, as well as protamine sulfate- and LPS-triggered foot process effacement [61].

Regarding the supportive function of synaptopodin on the actin cytoskeleton, this protein molecule not only constitutes a linkage to the actin cytoskeleton but remains vital for stress fiber synthesis in podocytes [62, 63]. Despite the previously presumed usefulness of calcineurin inhibitors, like cyclosporine A (CsA) and FK506 in the treatment of INS given their immunosuppressive effects on T cells, the mediatory role of calcineurin on synaptopodin degradation via induction of protease cathepsin L is well established; interestingly, CsA shields synaptopodin from cathepsin L-mediated breakdown, thereby maintaining the integrity of the actin cytoskeleton [64].

Finally, the regulatory activity of endocytic proteins in the actin cytoskeleton is confirmed by recent findings of possible therapeutic benefits of Bis-T-23-induced dynamin oligomerization and actin polymerization for nephrotic syndrome [65]. In fact, some researchers have shown that the GTPase dynamin is important for podocyte physiology [66]. In proteinuric kidney disease, induction of cytoplasmic cathepsin L results in degradation of dynamin, ending up with disruption of the actin cytoskeleton and proteinuria. Again, the modulating effect of dynamin on the actin cytoskeleton is related to the stabilization of the glomerulus. Thus, based on the beneficial activity of Bis-T-23 to kidney health in various models of chronic kidney disease (CKD) through the formation of actin-dependent oligomers of dynamin and polymers of actin, dynamin has been regarded as a possible therapeutic target for the management of CKD [67]. Better still, the recognition of dynamin as one of the vital and autonomous regulators of focal adhesion maturation suggests a molecular mechanism which underpins the beneficial effect of Bis-T-23 on podocyte physiology [67]. The efficacy of some of the therapeutic agents currently used in clinical practice and in experimental animal models is summarized in **Table 1**.

4. Conclusion

Significant progress has now been made in unraveling the complex molecular mechanisms and pathways responsible for maintaining podocyte health and thus the structural and functional integrity of the glomerular filtration barrier. Podocyte injury is now believed to be the basic pathology in childhood INS. As a podocytopathy, disruption of the podocyte architecture eventually results in the massive proteinuria seen in the syndrome. Consequently, several novel therapeutic targets have been proposed and successfully demonstrated, raising hopes for novel pharmacologic agents which could be useful in treating the disorder.

Author details

Samuel N. Uwaezuoke[1,2]

1 College of Medicine, University of Nigeria, Ituku-Ozalla Enugu Campus, Nigeria

2 Pediatric Nephrology Firm, University of Nigeria Teaching Hospital, Enugu, Nigeria

*Address all correspondence to: snuwaezuoke@yahoo.com; samuel.uwaezuoke@unn.edu.ng

References

[1] Eddy AA, Symons JM. Nephrotic syndrome in childhood. Lancet. 2003;**362**:629-639

[2] Churg J, Habib R, White RH. Pathology of the nephrotic syndrome in children a report for the International Study of Kidney Disease in children. Lancet. 1970;**760**:1299-1302

[3] Doe JY, Funk M, Mengel M, Doehring E, Ehrich JHH. Nephrotic syndrome in African children: Lack of evidence for 'tropical nephrotic syndrome'. Nephrology, Dialysis, Transplantation. 2006;**21**:672-676. DOI: 10.1093/ndt/gfi297

[4] Satgé P, Habib R, Quenum C, Boisson ME, Niang I. Particularité. du syndrome ne'phrotique chez l'enfant au Senegal. Ann Pe'diat. 1970;**17**:382-393

[5] Asinobi AO, Ademola AD, Okolo CA, Yaria JO. Trends in the histopathology of childhood nephrotic syndrome in Ibadan Nigeria: Preponderance of idiopathic focal segmental glomerulosclerosis. BMC Nephrology. 2015;**16**:213. DOI: 10.1186/s12882-015-0208-0

[6] Obiagwu PN, Aliyu A, Atanda AT. Nephrotic syndrome among children in Kano: A clinicopathological study. Nigerian Journal of Clinical Practice. 2014;**17**:370-374. DOI: 10.4103/1119-3077.130247

[7] Uwaezuoke SN, Okafor HU, Eneh CI, Odetunde OI. The triggers and patterns of relapse in childhood idiopathic nephrotic syndrome: A retrospective, descriptive study in a tertiary hospital, south-east Nigeria. Journal of Clinical Nephrology and Research. 2016;**3**(1):1032

[8] Asinobi AO, Gbadegesin RA, Adeyemo AA. The predominance of membrano-proliferative glomerulonephritis in childhood nephrotic syndrome in Ibadan. West African Journal of Medicine. 1999;**18**:203-206

[9] Kaneko K, Tsuji S, Kimata T, et al. Pathogenesis of childhood idiopathic nephrotic syndrome: A paradigm shift from T-cells to podocytes. World Journal of Pediatrics. 2015;**11**:21-28. DOI: 10.1007/s12519-015-0003-9

[10] Uwaezuoke SN. Pathogenesis of idiopathic nephrotic syndrome in children: Molecular mechanisms and therapeutic implications. Integrative Molecular Medicine. 2015;**3**:484-487. DOI: 10.15761/IMM.1000192

[11] Schönenberger E, Ehrich JH, Haller H, Schiffer M. The podocyte as a direct target of immunosuppressive agents. Nephrology, Dialysis, Transplantation. 2011;**26**:18-24. DOI: 10.1093/ndt/gfq617

[12] Uwaezuoke SN. Steroid-sensitive nephrotic syndrome in children: Triggers of relapse and evolving hypotheses on pathogenesis. Italian Journal of Pediatrics. 2015;**41**:19. DOI: 10.1186/s13052-015-0123-9

[13] Drenckhahn D, Franke RP. Ultrastructural organization of contractile and cytoskeletal proteins in glomerular podocytes of chicken, rat and man. Laboratory Investigation. 1988;**59**:673-682

[14] Mundel P, Kriz W. Structure and function of podocytes: An update. Anatomy and Embryology. 1995;**192**:385-397

[15] Adler S. Characterization of glomerular epithelial cell matrix receptors. The American Journal of Pathology. 1992;**141**:571-578

[16] Kriedberg JA, Donovan MJ, Goldstein SL, Rennke H, Shepherd K,

Jones RC, et al. Alpha 3 beta 1 integrin has a crucial role in kidney and lung organogenesis. Development. 1996;**122**:3537-3547

[17] Raats CJ, van Den Born J, Baker MA, et al. Expression of agrin, dystroglycan, and utrophin in normal renal tissue and in experimental glomerulopathies. The American Journal of Pathology. 2000;**156**:1749-1765. DOI: 10.1016/S0002-9440(10)65046-8

[18] Endlich K, Kriz W, Witzgall R. Update in podocyte biology. Current Opinion in Nephrology and Hypertension. 2001;**10**:331-340

[19] Tryggvason K, Wartiovaara J. Molecular basis of glomerular permselectivity. Current Opinion in Nephrology and Hypertension. 2001;**10**:543-549

[20] Holzman LB, St John PL, Kovari IA, et al. Nephrin localizes to the slit pore of the glomerular epithelial cell. Kidney International. 1999;**56**:1481-1491

[21] Schwarz K, Simons M, Reiser J, et al. Podocin, a raft-associated component of the glomerular slit diaphragm, interacts with CD2AP and nephrin. The Journal of Clinical Investigation. 2001;**108**:1621-1629. DOI: 10.1172/JCI12849

[22] Inoue T, Yaoita E, Kurihara H, et al. FAT is a component of glomerular slit diaphragms. Kidney International. 2001;**59**:1003-1012

[23] Mundel P, Gilbert P, Kriz W. Podocytes in glomerulus of rat kidney express a characteristic 44KD protein. The Journal of Histochemistry and Cytochemistry. 1991;**39**:1047-1056

[24] Patrie KM, Drescher AJ, Welihinda A, Mundel P, Margolis B. Interaction of two actin-binding proteins, synaptopodin and alpha-actinin-4, with the tight junction protein MAGI-1. The Journal of Biological Chemistry. 2002;**277**:30183-30190

[25] Tian X, Ishibe S. Targeting the podocyte cytoskeleton: From pathogenesis to therapy in proteinuric kidney disease. Nephrology, Dialysis, Transplantation. 2016;**31**:1577-1583. DOI: 10.1093/ndt/gfw021

[26] Ma H, Togawa A, Soda K, et al. Inhibition of podocyte FAK protects against proteinuria and foot process effacement. Journal of the American Society of Nephrology. 2010;**21**:1145-1156. DOI: 10.1681/ASN.2009090991

[27] Donoviel DB, Freed DD, Vogel H, et al. Proteinuria and perinatal lethality in mice lacking NEPH1, a novel protein with homology to NEPHRIN. Molecular and Cellular Biology. 2001;**21**:4829-4836. DOI: 10.1128/MCB.21.14.4829-4836.2001

[28] Shaw AS, Miner JH. CD2-associated protein and the kidney. Current Opinion in Nephrology and Hypertension. 2001;**10**:19-22

[29] Boute N, Gribouval O, Roselli S, et al. NPHS2, encoding the glomerular protein podocin, is mutated in autosomal recessive steroid-resistant nephrotic syndrome. Nature Genetics. 2000;**24**:349-354. DOI: 10.1038/74166

[30] Patrakka J, Tryggvason K. Nephrin: A unique structural and signaling protein of the kidney filter. Trends in Molecular Medicine. 2007;**13**:396-403. DOI: 10.1016/j.molmed.2007.06.006

[31] Yuan H, Takeuchi E, Salant DJ. Podocyte slit-diaphragm protein nephrin is linked to the actin cytoskeleton. American Journal of Physiology. Renal Physiology. 2002;**282**:F585-F591. DOI: 10.1152/ajprenal.00290.2001

[32] Lehtonen S, Zhao F, Lehtonen E. CD2-associated protein directly

interacts with the actin cytoskeleton. American Journal of Physiology. Renal Physiology. 2002;**283**:F734-F743. DOI: 10.1152/ajprenal.00312.2001

[33] Somlo S, Mundel P. Getting a foothold in nephrotic syndrome. Nature Genetics. 2000;**24**:333-335. DOI: 10.1038/74139

[34] Andrews PM. Investigations of cytoplasmic contractile and cytoskeletal elements in the kidney glomerulus. Kidney International. 1981;**20**:549-562

[35] Mundel P, Heid HW, Mundel TM, et al. Synaptopodin: An actin-associated protein in telencephalic dendrites and renal podocytes. The Journal of Cell Biology. 1997;**139**:193-204

[36] Smoyer WE, Mundel P, Gupta A, Welsh MJ. Podocyte alpha-actinin induction precedes foot process effacement in experimental nephrotic syndrome. The American Journal of Physiology. 1997;**273**:F150-F157

[37] Srivastava T, Garola RE, Whiting JM, Alon US. Synaptopodin expression in idiopathic nephrotic syndrome of childhood. Kidney International. 2001;**59**:118-125. DOI: 10.1046/j.1523-1755.2001.00472.x

[38] Kerjaschki D, Sharkey DJ, Farquhar MG. Identification and characterization of podocalyxin—The major sialoprotein of the renal glomerular epithelial cell. The Journal of Cell Biology. 1984;**98**:1591-1596

[39] Kavoura E, Gakiopoulou H, Paraskevakou H, et al. Immunohistochemical evaluation of podocalyxin expression in glomerulopathies associated with nephrotic syndrome. Human Pathology. 2011;**42**:227-235. DOI: 10.1016/j.humpath.2010.05.028

[40] Pozzi A, Jarad G, Moeckel GW, et al. Beta1 integrin expression by podocytes is required to maintain glomerular structural integrity. Developmental Biology. 2008;**316**:288-301. DOI: 10.1016/j.ydbio.2008.01.022

[41] Kanasaki K, Kanda Y, Palmsten K, et al. Integrin beta1-mediated matrix assembly and signaling are critical for the normal development and function of the kidney glomerulus. Developmental Biology. 2008;**313**:584-593

[42] Wei C, Möller CC, Altintas MM, et al. Modification of kidney barrier function by the urokinase receptor. Nature Medicine. 2008;**14**:55-63. DOI: 10.1038/nm1696

[43] Wei C, El Hindi S, Li J, et al. Circulating urokinase receptor as a cause of focal segmental glomerulosclerosis. Nature Medicine. 2011;**17**:952-960. DOI: 10.1038/nm.2411

[44] Lin Y, Rao J, Zha XL, Xu H. Angiopoietin-like 3 induces podocyte F-actin rearrangement through integrin α (V) β_3/FAK/PI3K pathway-mediated Rac1 activation. BioMed Research International. vol 2013; Article ID 135608, 8 pages. DOI: 10.1155/2013/135608

[45] Pertz O, Hodgson L, Klemke RL, Hahn KM. Spatiotemporal dynamics of RhoA activity in migrating cells. Nature. 2006;**440**:1069-1072. DOI: 10.1038/nature04665

[46] Heasman SJ, Ridley AJ. Mammalian Rho GTPases: New insights into their functions from in vivo studies. Nature Reviews. Molecular Cell Biology. 2008;**9**:690-701. DOI: 10.1038/nrm2476

[47] Babelova A, Jansen F, Sander K, et al. Activation of Rac-1 and RhoA contributes to podocyte injury in chronic kidney disease. PLoS One. 2013;**8**:(11):e80328. DOI: 10.1371/journal.pone.0080328

[48] Hidaka T, Suzuki Y, Yamashita M, et al. Amelioration of crescentic glomerulonephritis by RhoA kinase inhibitor, Fasudil, through podocyte protection and prevention of leukocyte migration. The American Journal of Pathology. 2008;**172**:603-614

[49] Shikawa Y, Nishikimi T, Akimoto K, et al. Long-term administration of rho-kinase inhibitor ameliorates renal damage in malignant hypertensive rats. Hypertension. 2006;**47**:1075-1083. DOI: 10.1161/01.HYP.0000221605.94532.71

[50] Sun GP, Kohno M, Guo P, et al. Involvements of Rho-kinase and TGF-beta pathways in aldosterone-induced renal injury. Journal of the American Society of Nephrology. 2006;**17**:2193-2201. DOI: 10.1681/ASN. 2005121375

[51] Wang L, Ellis MJ, Gomez JA, et al. Mechanisms of the proteinuria induced by Rho GTPases. Kidney International. 2012;**81**:1075-1085. DOI: 10.1038/ki.2011.472

[52] Borza CM, Su Y, Chen X, et al. Inhibition of integrin α2β1 ameliorates glomerular injury. Journal of the American Society of Nephrology. 2012;**23**:1027-1038

[53] George B, Verma R, Soofi AA, Garg P, Zhang J, Park TJ, et al. Crk1/2-dependent signaling is necessary for podocyte foot process spreading in mouse models of glomerular disease. The Journal of Clinical Investigation. 2012;**122**:674-692. DOI: 10.1172/JCI60070

[54] Yu CC, Fornoni A, Weins A, et al. Abatacept in B7-1-positive proteinuric kidney disease. The New England Journal of Medicine. 2013;**369**:2416-2423. DOI: 10.1056/NEJMoa1304572

[55] Abramowitz J, Birnbaumer L. Physiology and pathophysiology of canonical transient receptor potential channels. The FASEB Journal. 2009;**23**:297-328. DOI: 10.1096/fj.08-119495

[56] Goel M, Sinkins WG, Zuo CD, Estacion M, Schilling WP. Identification and localization of TRPC channels in the rat kidney. American Journal of Physiology. Renal Physiology. 2006;**290**:F1241-F1252. DOI: 10.1152/ajprenal.00376.2005

[57] Dryer SE, Reiser J. TRPC6 channels and their binding partners in podocytes: Role in glomerular filtration and pathophysiology. American Journal of Physiology. Renal Physiology. 2010;**299**:689-701. DOI: 10.1152/ajprenal. 00298.2010

[58] Kalwa H, Storch U, Demleitner J, et al. Phospholipase C epsilon (PLCε) induced TRPC6 activation: A common but redundant mechanism in primary podocytes. Journal of Cellular Physiology. 2015;**230**:1389-1399. DOI: 10.1002/jcp.24883

[59] Ilatovskaya DV, Levchenko V, Ryan RP, Cowley AW Jr, Staruschenko A. NSAIDs acutely inhibit TRPC channels in freshly isolated rat glomeruli. Biochemical and Biophysical Research Communications. 2011;**408**:242-247. DOI: 10.1016/j.bbrc.2011.04.005

[60] Kim EY, Alvarez-Baron CP, Dryer SE. Canonical transient receptor potential channel (TRPC) 3 and TRPC6 associate with large-conductance Ca2+-activated K+ (BKCa) channels: Role in BKCa trafficking to the surface of cultured podocytes. Molecular Pharmacology. 2009;**75**:466-477. DOI: 10.1124/mol.108.051912

[61] Schaldecker T, Kim S, Tarabanis C, et al. Inhibition of the TRPC5 ion channel protects the kidney filter. The Journal of Clinical Investigation. 2013;**123**:5298-5309. DOI: 10.1172/JCI71165

[62] Asanuma K, Kim K, Oh J, et al. Synaptopodin regulates the actin-bundling activity of alpha-actinin in an isoform-specific manner. The Journal of Clinical Investigation. 2005;**115**:1188-1198. DOI: 10.1172/JCI23371

[63] Asanuma K, Yanagida-Asanuma E, Faul C, et al. Synaptopodin orchestrates actin organization and cell motility via regulation of RhoA signaling. Nature Cell Biology. 2006;**8**:485-491. DOI: 10.1038/ncb1400

[64] Faul C, Donnelly M, Merscher-Gomez S, et al. The actin cytoskeleton of kidney podocytes is a direct target of the antiproteinuric effect of cyclosporine A. Nature Medicine. 2008;**14**:931-938. DOI: 10.1038/nm.1857

[65] Schiffer M, Teng B, Gu C, et al. Pharmacological targeting of actin-dependent dynamin oligomerization ameliorates chronic kidney disease in diverse animal models. Nature Medicine. 2015;**21**:601-609. DOI: 10.1038/nm.3843

[66] Sever S, Altintas MM, Nankoe SR, et al. Proteolytic processing of dynamin by cytoplasmic cathepsin L is a mechanism for proteinuric kidney disease. The Journal of Clinical Investigation. 2007;**117**:2095-2104. DOI: 10.1172/JCI32022

[67] Gu C, Lee HW, Garborcauskas G, Reiser J, Gupta V, Sever S. Dynamin autonomously regulates podocyte focal adhesion maturation. Journal of the American Society of Nephrology. 2017;**28**:446-451. DOI: 10.1681/ASN.2016010008

[68] Uwaezuoke SN. Childhood idiopathic nephrotic syndrome as a podocytopathy: Potential therapeutic targets. Journal of Clinical Nephrology and Research. 2017;**4**(4):1071

Section 3

Membranous Nephropathy

Chapter 4

Membranous Nephropathy

Bhadran Bose, Sunil V. Badve, Vivekanand Jha, Chen Au Peh and David Johnson

Abstract

Membranous nephropathy (MN) is a glomerular disease that is the leading cause of nephrotic syndrome in non-diabetic Caucasian adults. MN is most often primary (idiopathic) and the remaining is secondary to systemic disease or exposure to infection or drugs. The majority of patients with MN have circulating antibodies to the podocyte antigens phospholipase A_2 receptor (PLA2R) (70%) and thrombospondin type-1 domain-containing 7A (THSD7A) (3–5%). Immunologic remission (depletion of PLA2R antibodies) often precedes and may predict clinical remission. Untreated, about one-third of patients undergo spontaneous remission, one-third have persistent proteinuria but maintain kidney function and the remaining one-third will develop end stage kidney failure. All patients with idiopathic MN should be treated with conservative care from the time of diagnosis to minimise proteinuria. Immunosuppressive therapy is traditionally reserved for patients who have persistent nephrotic-range proteinuria despite conservative care. Immunosuppressive agents for primary MN include combination of corticosteroids/alkylating agent or calcineurin inhibitors and rituximab. This chapter will review the epidemiology, diagnosis and treatment of MN, particularly focusing on idiopathic MN.

Keywords: membranous nephropathy, PLA2R antibody, cytotoxic agents, calcineurin inhibitor, rituximab

1. Introduction

Idiopathic membranous nephropathy (MN) remains the leading cause of nephrotic syndrome in Caucasian adults and one of the most common primary glomerular diseases to progress to end-stage kidney disease (ESKD) [1, 2]. Secondary MN is associated with autoimmune diseases (e.g., systemic lupus erythematosus), infections (e.g., hepatitis B and C), medications (e.g., nonsteroidal anti-inflammatory drugs, D-penicillamine, gold), and neoplasias [3]. As idiopathic and secondary forms have similar clinical presentations, the designation of idiopathic is made only after ruling out secondary causes by a careful history, physical examination, and laboratory evaluation. This chapter will primarily focus on idiopathic MN.

2. Epidemiology

MN accounts for 20–30% of cases of nephrotic syndrome in Caucasian adults [4, 5]. Although the disease affects patients of all ages, all ethnicities and both sexes, it is more common in white men [4, 6]. MN has a peak incidence during the fourth and fifth decades of life, and is relatively uncommon in patients aged under 20 years [4, 6]. The incidence of ESKD is about 35% at 10 years [7].

3. Pathogenesis

In the past decade, the understanding of the pathogenesis of idiopathic MN has significantly improved. In 2009, phospholipase A_2 receptor (PLA2R) was identified as the major antigen responsible for autoantibody binding in idiopathic MN [8]. PLA2R is a transmembrane receptor that is highly expressed in glomerular podocytes and anti-PLA2R (typically of IgG4 subtype) was initially identified in 70% of patients with idiopathic MN [8]. Subsequent studies from various cohorts have shown that PLA2R antibodies are positive in 50–80% of patients with idiopathic MN [4, 6, 9–12]. PLA2R antibodies are uncommon in patients with MN associated with malignancies [13, 14]. PLA2R antibody has been reported in hepatitis-B associated membranous nephropathy [15] and also in hepatitis-C associated membranous nephropathy [14]. In genetic studies, there was association with HLA-DQA1 risk alleles [16, 17] and PLA2R1 alleles [16]. Furthermore, the presence of HLA DQA1*05:01 and DQB1*02:01 alleles are associated with higher PLA2R antibody levels [18].

PLA2R is a 180-kDa membrane receptor with a large extracellular region comprising 10 distinct globular domains, including a cysteine-rich domain, a fibronectin type II domain, and eight distinct C-type lectin domains (CTLD1–8) [19]. Each domain is separated by a small linker sequence of <10 amino acids. CysR is the immunodominant epitope for PLA2R [20]. Epitope spreading refers to the development of immune responses to endogenous epitopes secondary to the release of self-antigens during a chronic autoimmune or inflammatory response. In MN, epitope-spreading starts with the cysteine-rich domain then extends to CTLD1, CTLD7 or other nearby regions. This results in an augmented immune response through heightened antibody diversity. In a study of 69 patients with MN from five French centres, Seitz-Polski et al. demonstrated that higher anti-PLA2R antibody titres and serum reactivity to CTLD1 and/or CTLD7 in addition to the cysteine-rich domain were associated with a higher rate of kidney failure [21].

A second IgG4 auto-antibody against thrombospondin type-1 domain-containing 7A (THSD7A) was identified in a smaller number of patients with MN. THSD7A, like PLA2R, is also a protein highly expressed in podocytes and was identified in European and North American patients with anti-PLA2R-negative idiopathic MN but not in healthy controls or patients with other glomerular diseases [22]. It occurred in 2–5% of all patients with idiopathic membranous nephropathy, which corresponded to 8–14% of patients who were seronegative for anti-PLA_2R antibodies. A recent meta-analysis of 10 studies involving 4121 patients showed that the prevalence of THSD7A was low at 3% (95% CI 2–4%) of all patients with idiopathic MN, which corresponded to 10% (95% CI 6–15%) of anti-PLA2R antibody negative patients [23]. However, this meta-analysis was limited by a limited number of studies and small sample size. This meta-analysis also showed that cancer may be more common in patients with THSD7A antibodies and the incidence varied from 6 to 25%. Further studies to elucidate the role of THSD7A as a marker of prognosis and response to therapy are required.

Antibodies against both PLA2R and THSD7A can coexist but only in 1% of cases [24].

4. Pathology

Despite the availability of anti-PLA2R antibody, kidney biopsy remains the standard of care in diagnosing MN. In early MN, glomeruli may appear normal by light microscopy. However, with time, the glomerular basement membrane thickens and there is formation of subepithelial "spikes" of basement membrane on the outer surface of the capillary wall. These "spikes" are more apparent with silver methenamine staining (**Figure 1**). Immunofluorescence microscopy reveals diffuse, uniform, finely granular deposits of IgG4 along the outer surfaces of capillary walls (**Figure 2**). Complement components, including C3, C4d and C5b-9, are also

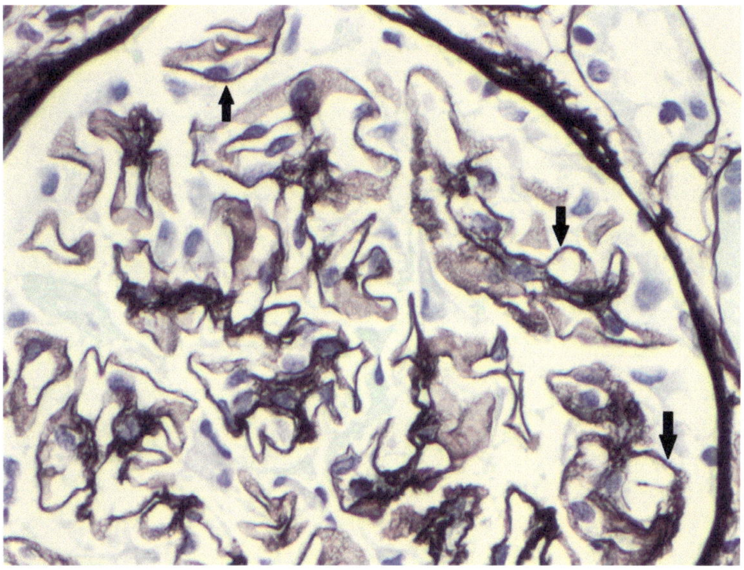

Figure 1.
Glomerulus showing thickening of glomerular basement membrane and subepithelial "spikes" (see arrowhead) in MN (silver-methamine stain).

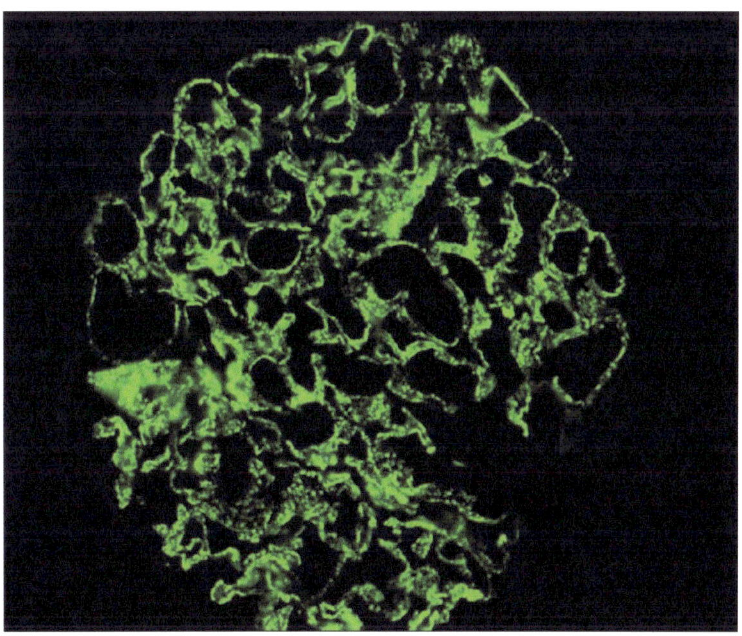

Figure 2.
Immunofluorescence showing diffuse fine granular distribution pattern of immunoglobulin G (IgG) along the glomerular basement membrane.

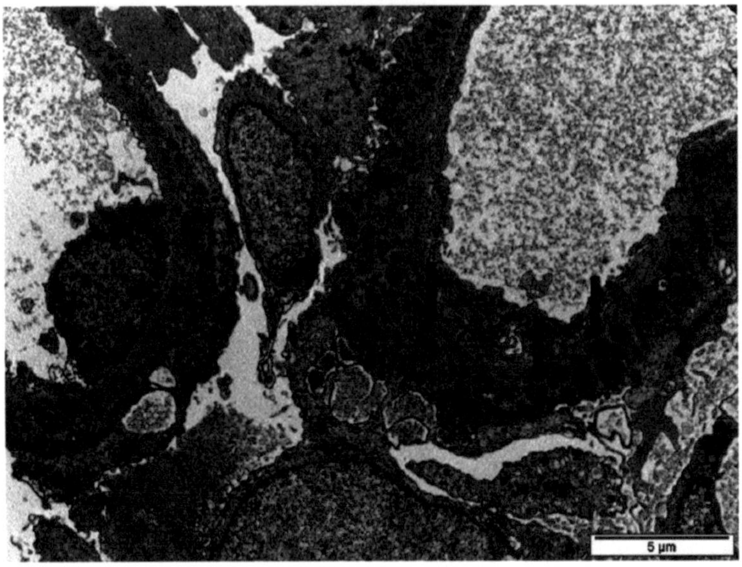

Figure 3.
Electron microscopy showing diffuse subepithelial electron dense deposits (see arrowheads) in MN.

commonly present, but not C1q. The antigens, PLA2R and THSD7A, co-localise with IgG4 in most patients with idiopathic MN.

Electron microscopy shows diffuse subepithelial electron-dense deposits and also glomerular basement membrane thickening (**Figure 3**). The deposits are gradually incorporated within new glomerular basement membrane and become more electron-lucent as they are resorbed before eventually disappearing in patients following the development of complete remission (CR).

5. Clinical manifestations

At presentation, 60–70% of patients will have nephrotic syndrome [25, 26]. The remaining one-third is presented with sub nephrotic-range proteinuria (<3.5 g/day) [27]. Microscopic hematuria also occurs in approximately one-third of patients; however, macroscopic hematuria is unusual and should prompt consideration of alternative diagnoses [28]. Hypertension and moderate-to-severe kidney failure occur in a minority of patients and tend to occur more commonly in older individuals [29]. Dyslipidaemia is common and venous thromboembolism has been reported to occur in approximately 7% [30].

6. Natural history

MN is a chronic disease, with spontaneous remission and relapses. There is great variability in the rate of disease progression, and the natural course is difficult to assess [31–33]. Spontaneous remissions are said to occur in up to 30% of cases. The proportion of patients going into spontaneous remission is much lower when patients have higher grades of proteinuria or high anti-PLA2R antibody titre (>85 RU/mL) at presentation [34]. The remaining two-thirds of patients who do not undergo spontaneous remission either have persistent proteinuria with stable kidney function long-term or will progress to kidney failure. Even patients who do not progress but remain nephrotic are at an increased risk for life-threatening thromboembolic and cardiovascular events [30, 35, 36]. A rapid decline in kidney function should raise the possibility of a superimposed condition, such as interstitial nephritis, renal vein thrombosis or acute tubular necrosis due to sepsis in an immunocompromised patient.

7. Predicting factors

Many individual factors, such as advanced age, male sex, degree of kidney impairment on presentation, degree of chronicity in the kidney biopsy (e.g., degree of interstitial fibrosis, tubular atrophy, vascular damage and glomerulosclerosis), degree of proteinuria and anti-PLA2R antibody titre have all been reported to be predictors of prognosis and/or response to immunosuppressive therapy in patients with MN [34, 37]. Pei et al. observed a 47% higher risk of kidney disease progression in patients with proteinuria exceeding 4 g/24 hour for longer than 18 months and a 66% higher risk in patients with proteinuria exceeding 8 g/24 hour for more than 6 months [38]. Similarly, PLA_2R antibodies appear to correlate with disease activity, response to therapy and also prognosis [18, 34, 39, 40]. In particular, higher antibody levels are linked to a higher risk of declining kidney function, suggesting that these affected individuals may benefit from earlier initiation of immunosuppression [18]. Conversely, favourable outcomes have been shown in patients who are negative for anti-PLA_2R antibodies.

8. Response measurements

The best-accepted responses are improved kidney survival and CR of proteinuria. CR is defined as a urine protein excretion of <0.3 g/24 hour accompanied by a normal serum albumin concentration and normal serum creatinine [41]. Partial remission (PR) has been also recognised as a positive outcome and is defined as urine protein excretion of <3.5 g/24 hour or reduced by at least 50% from peak values accompanied by an improvement or normalisation of the serum albumin concentration and stable serum creatinine [41]. Approximately 30% of MN cases will relapse subsequent to a CR [42]. The great majority who do, however, will relapse to sub-nephrotic-range proteinuria and will have stable long-term function [42]. A review of 350 nephrotic patients with MN found that the 10-year kidney survival was 100% in the CR group, 90% in the PR group, and 45% in the no-remission group [43]. Respective rates of glomerular filtration rate decline were -0.12 ± 0.40, -0.17 ± 0.50 and -0.86 ± 1.08 mL/minute/month, such that the attainment of CR or PR independently predicted a much more favourable kidney function prognosis [43]. In patients who are anti-PLA2R antibody positive, reduction in circulating antibody titre precedes clinical remission, and furthermore, persistence of antibody despite treatment is associated with clinical resistance [44]. Future definitions of remission of this disease may well incorporate elements of both clinical and serological remission.

9. Treatment

Based on the predictive factors described above, patients can be rationally assigned to either conservative (non-immunosuppressive) therapy or immunosuppressive therapy.

10. Conservative therapy

Conservative therapy includes controlling oedema, dietary protein intake, blood pressure, and hyperlipidaemia. MN patients develop significant oedema and to control the oedema, loop diuretic is the mainstay of treatment along with low-salt diet. High salt diet intake, apart from worsening the oedema, can also significantly impair the beneficial effects of renin-angiotensin blockade, which are one of the key components of conservative therapy. A normal dietary protein intake (0.75–1.0 g/kg/day) is usually recommended. A recent meta-analysis including 44,989 participants showed more intensive blood pressure-lowering (mean blood pressure levels of 133/76 mm Hg, compared with 140/81 mm Hg in the less intensive treatment group) achieved a relative risk reduction of albuminuria by 10% [45]. Anti-proteinuric agents, such as angiotensin converting enzyme inhibitors (ACEi) or angiotensin receptor blockers (ARBs), should be used as first-line antihypertensive agents [46, 47]. In patients with lower levels of proteinuria (<4 g/24 hour), treatment with an ACEi or an ARB may be sufficient to reduce proteinuria to sub-nephrotic levels thereby appreciably mitigating kidney and cardiovascular risks. However, in patients with higher degrees of proteinuria, the use of these medications alone is unlikely to result in a substantial reduction in proteinuria or preservation of kidney function [48].

Statins should be prescribed to control hypercholesterolaemia and attenuate the heightened cardiovascular risk observed in patients with MN [49].

Patients with severe nephrotic syndrome are at increased risk of thromboembolic complications. Lionaki et al. reported that clinically apparent venous thromboembolism occurred in 7% of patients with MN and the risk was higher if the serum albumin was below 2.8 g/dL [30]. In a retrospective review of MN patients with nephrotic range proteinuria, use of prophylactic anticoagulation has been shown to be associated with a reduction in fatal thromboembolic episodes and benefits of anticoagulation outweigh the risk of bleeding [50]. In general, MN patients who are severely nephrotic (proteinuria >10 g/24 hour and serum albumin of <2.5 g/dL) should be considered for anticoagulation [30].

11. Immunosuppressive therapy

Several treatment strategies using immunosuppressive therapy have been shown to be successful in reducing proteinuria in MN [51]. Based on their risk factor profiles, patients are grouped into low, medium and high-risk categories.

12. Treatment of low-risk patients

Patients in the low-risk group are categorised by a <5% risk of kidney disease progression over 5 years of observation. Patients in this group would have normal kidney function and proteinuria of ≤4 g/24 hours over a 6-month observation period. Evidence to support this approach comes from published validation studies [43, 52]. Such patients therefore do well with a conservative treatment approach, as outlined above [53].

13. Treatment of medium-risk patients

Patients in this group have preserved renal function and daily urinary protein excretion rates of 4–8 g/24 hours which continue unabated following a 6 month period of conservative therapy. These patients warrant immunosuppressive therapy with one or more of the following options:

13.1 Corticosteroid monotherapy

An early collaborative randomized study of 72 adult patients with idiopathic nephrotic syndrome demonstrated that a 2–3 month course of high-dose alternate-day prednisone when compared to placebo resulted in a significant reduction in progression to kidney failure but there was no effect on the degree of proteinuria. Ten of the 38 placebo-treated and one of the 34 prednisone-treated patient were in renal failure (creatinine more than 5 mg/dL [440 μmol/L]) or dead ($p < 0.02$) [54]. A subsequent prospective randomised study comparing a 6-month course of alternate day prednisone (45 mg/m^2) or no specific treatment in 158 patients with idiopathic MN showed no significant benefit of corticosteroid treatment alone in either induction of remission or preservation of kidney function over a mean follow-up period of 48 months [55]. Hence, corticosteroid monotherapy have been shown to be ineffective inducing remission in patients with MN.

13.2 Cytotoxic agents combined with corticosteroids

A number of randomised trials have suggested that alternating monthly regimen of steroids and cytotoxic agents is more likely to induce CR of nephrotic syndrome, and halt disease progression compared to no therapy or corticosteroids alone. The first study by Ponticelli's group compared the effects of corticosteroids alternating monthly with chlorambucil to conservative treatment in 67 adult patients with MN [56]. The regimen was given over a 6-month period. It consists of 1 g of intravenous methylprednisolone (MTP)/day for first 3 days of months 1, 3 and 5 followed by 27 days of oral methylprednisolone 0.5 mg/kg/day for the remainder of the month. In the alternating months (months 2, 4 and 6), chlorambucil 0.2 mg/kg/day is used instead of corticosteroids. Compared with controls, patients in the intervention group experienced higher rates of CR or PR (72 vs. 30%, $p = 0.001$) and significantly better preserved kidney function at 1 year ($p = 0.011$) and 2 years ($p < 0.0001$). After 10 years of follow-up, patients treated with combination therapy had a 92% probability of kidney survival compared with 60% in the control group ($p = 0.004$), and the probability of achieving a CR or PR was 83% in the treatment group, and only 38% in the controls ($p = 0.000$) [57]. A second study by the same group, compared the original chlorambucil regimen (45 patients) as described above to MTP pulses plus steroid alone for 6 months (47 patients) [58]. Compared to the steroids alone regimen, treatment with the chlorambucil regimen resulted in higher proportions of patients without nephrotic syndrome at 3 years (66 vs. 40%, $p = 0.011$), although the result was no longer statistically significant by 4 years (62 vs. 42%, $p = 0.102$) chlorambucil-treated patients also had longer mean ratios of months in remission (0.52 vs. 0.31, $p = 0.008$) [58]. In a third study from the same investigators, patients were enrolled in a 6-month study comparing corticosteroids (1 gm of intravenous MTP day for first 3 days of months 1, 3 and 5 followed by 27 days of oral methylprednisolone 0.5 mg/kg/day for the remainder of the month) alternating monthly with either chlorambucil (0.2 mg/kg/day) or oral cyclophosphamide (2.5 mg/kg/day) in months 2, 4 and 6 [59]. No significant differences were observed between the two groups with respect to remission rate (CR or PR) at 1 year (82 vs. 93%, respectively, $p = 0.116$), subsequent relapse rate (31 vs. 25%, or changes in proteinuria or reciprocal serum creatinine over time.

In an open-label, parallel-arm, randomised controlled trial, Jha and colleagues compared the effects of alternating monthly prednisolone and cyclophosphamide for 6 months versus conservative treatment (salt restriction, blood pressure control and diuretic therapy) on remission, kidney disease progression and quality of life in adult patients with MN and nephrotic syndrome [60]. Compared with controls, those who received cyclophosphamide and steroids were more likely to achieve remission (72 vs. 35%, $p < 0.001$) and have better kidney survival, defined as not experiencing doubling of serum creatinine, dialysis or death (79 vs. 44%, $p = 0.0006$) [60]. They also had higher mean quality of life scores at 10 years, as measured by a visual analogue scale (7.31 ± 0.76 vs. 6.61 ± 1.08, $p < 0.01$). Infectious complications were similar between the groups.

Adverse effects associated with these agents, particularly infertility and malignancy, are the major drawbacks of cytotoxics combined with corticosteroids. The risk of malignancy is not increased for patients treated with cumulative cyclophosphamide doses of up to 36 g but increases significantly thereafter [61].

13.3 Cyclosporine

Early uncontrolled studies of cyclosporine (CSA) suggested an initial benefit but a high relapse rate [62, 63]. In the first single-blind randomised controlled study, 51 patients with steroid-resistant MN were treated with low-dose prednisone (0.15 mg/kg/day up to a maximum dose of 15 mg and reduced after 26 weeks by thirds at 4-week intervals) plus CsA (3.5 mg/kg/day in two divided doses and aiming for a trough level between 125 and 225 µg/L) and compared to patients treated with placebo plus prednisone (similar dose to treatment arm) [64]. At the end of 26 weeks of treatment, 75% of patients (21 of 28) in the CsA group versus only 22% of patients (5 of 23) in the controls had achieved a CR or PR ($P < 0.001$). Relapses occurred in about 40% of patients within 1 year of discontinuation of CsA treatment. In an observational study of 36 adults with idiopathic MN and steroid-dependent or -resistant nephrotic syndrome treated with CsA (5.54 ± 0.81 mg/kg/day), the German Cyclosporine in Nephrotic Syndrome Study Group reported that prolonging CsA treatment (>1 year) resulted in a higher (34% CR at 1 year) and more sustained rate of remission [65]. Prolonged low-dose CsA (~1.5 mg/kg/day) could be considered for long-term maintenance of patients who achieve CR or PR, especially in patients at high risk of relapse [66]. However, this needs to be weighed against the risk of renal scarring from long-term exposure to CsA.

13.4 Tacrolimus

Tacrolimus is also a reasonable consideration for the treatment of MN. In an open-label, randomised controlled trial of tacrolimus versus conservative therapy in 48 patients with MN, normal kidney function and nephrotic syndrome from 13 Spanish centres, Praga et al. demonstrated that tacrolimus monotherapy resulted in a higher probability of remission (CR or PR) at 12 months (76 vs. 22%, $p < 0.001$) with shorter mean time to remission (61. vs. 11.3 months, $p = 0.003$) [67]. In patients with CR or PR at 18 months who subsequently had their tacrolimus withdrawn, 47% of patients experienced a relapse of nephrotic syndrome within a mean period of 4.2 months.

14. Treatment of high-risk patients

This group of patients is characterised by worsening kidney failure, extremely high anti-PLA2R antibodies or persistent high proteinuria (≥8 g/day).

14.1 Corticosteroids

A prospective double-blind randomised controlled trial by the UK Medical Research assessed the medium-term effect of an 8-week course of high-dose prednisolone (100–150 mg on alternate day) in a high risk MN population [68]. A total of 103 patients with preserved kidney function (average creatinine clearance 88 ± 30 mL/minute) were randomised to the treatment group ($n = 52$) or to the control group ($n = 51$). At 36 months, there was no significant difference regarding the degree of proteinuria or loss of kidney function between the control and the treatment group.

14.2 Cytotoxic agents combined with corticosteroids

Another randomised controlled trial by the same group assessed whether immunosuppression preserved kidney function in patients with idiopathic MN and declining kidney function [69]. The study randomised patients to either combination of prednisolone and chlorambucil (intravenous methyl prednisolone 1 g per day for 3 consecutive days then oral prednisolone 0·5 mg/kg per day for 28 days during months 1, 3, and 5. During months 2, 4, and 6, patients received oral chlorambucil at a starting dose of 0·15 mg/kg per day) ($n = 33$) or CsA (12 months of CsA received a starting dose of 5 mg/kg per day, aiming for trough level of 100–200 μg/L) ($n = 37$) or supportive therapy alone ($n = 38$). The primary endpoint was a further 20% decline in Cockcroft-Gault estimated creatinine clearance and occurred less frequently in the prednisolone and chlorambucil group than in either the cyclosporin or supportive therapy groups (58 vs. 81 vs. 84%, respectively, $p = 0.003$). Serious adverse events were also most common in the prednisolone and chlorambucil group (52 vs. 46 vs. 29%, respectively).

14.3 Cyclosporine

So far, there has been only one controlled trial with CsA in patients with high-grade proteinuria and progressive kidney failure. In this study, patients with high risk features were randomly assigned to either CsA (3.5 mg/kg/day taken in two divided doses, and aiming for trough level between 110 and 170 μg/L) treatment (nine patients) or placebo (eight patients) for 12 months) [70]. The average creatinine clearance of these patients was 51 mL/minute/1.73 m^2 and they had an average daily urine protein excretion of 11.5 g/day. After 12 months, there was a significant improvement in renal function as measured by the change in slopes, being greater in the CsA versus placebo patients [70 vs. 7% improvement, mean difference 1.5 (95% CI 0.2–3.1)]. Proteinuria in the CsA group was reduced by an average of 4.5 g/day, where in the placebo group there was an increase of 0.7 g/day by month 3 ($p = 0.02$).

14.4 Mycophenolate mofetil

In a pilot study, Miller et al. treated 16 medium or high risk MN patients with 1.5–2 g/day of mycophenolate mofetil for a mean period of 8 months [71]. There were no significant changes in mean serum creatinine or albumin levels over the course of the study. Similar results were reported in a retrospective analysis of 17 patients with MN [72], in which treatment with mycophenolate mofetil for 12 months combined with steroids resulted in a 61% reduction of proteinuria. Kidney function improved in three of six patients with kidney failure.

Branten et al. reported 32 patients with MN and kidney insufficiency treated with mycophenolate mofetil (1 g twice a day) plus steroids (IV MTP 1 g for 3 consecutive days at the beginning of months 1, 3, and 5 and oral prednisone, 0.5 mg/kg every other day, for 6 months with subsequent tapering for 12 months) and compared the results with those obtained for 32 patients from a historic control group treated for the same period of time with oral cyclophosphamide (1.5 mg/kg/day) and steroids (similar steroid schedule to above) [73]. Overall, 21 mycophenolate-treated patients developed PR of proteinuria, six patients experienced at least 50% reduction in proteinuria, and five patients experienced no response. No significant differences were observed between the intervention and control groups at 12 months with respect to the occurrence of CR or PR (66 vs. 72%, respectively, $p = 0.30$) or adverse drug reactions (75 vs. 69%, $p = 0.60$), although relapse occurred more frequently in those who received mycophenolate mofetil (38 vs. 13%, $p < 0.01$).

14.5 Rituximab

In a pilot study of eight MN patients treated with four weekly courses of rituximab (375 mg/m^2), two achieved CR and three achieved PR by 12 months [74, 75]. Mean 24-hour urinary protein excretion rates fell by 66% from 8.6 to 3.0 g ($p < 0.005$). Kidney function remained stable in all patients. Adverse effects were reported as mild and included chills, fever and an anxiety reaction.

In another prospective open-label pilot trial, 15 patients with idiopathic MN and proteinuria of >4 g/24 hour despite conservative therapy for >3 months received two doses of rituximab (1 g) 2 weeks apart [76]. At 6 months, another two fortnightly doses of rituximab were administered to patients with measured 24-hour urinary protein excretion rates exceeding 3 g and total CD19$^+$ B-cell counts exceeding 15 cells/μL. Mean proteinuria levels decreased by 54% from 13.0 g/24 hour at baseline to 6.0 g/24 hour at 12 months. At 12 months, two patients achieved CR, six achieved PR, five did not respond and two progressed to ESKD. Rituximab was well-tolerated and was effective in reducing proteinuria in patients with idiopathic MN.

The Evaluate Rituximab Treatment for Idiopathic Membranous Nephropathy (GEMRITUX) study was a French multicentre, randomised, controlled trial which evaluated the efficacy of rituximab in inducing remission in medium- to high-risk patients with idiopathic membranous nephropathy [77]. Thirty-seven patients received both rituximab (375 mg/m^2 on days 1 and 8) and conservative therapy and 38 patients received conservative therapy alone. There was no significant difference in remission rates at 6 months (35.1% in rituximab group compared to 21.1% in conservative group, $p = 0.21$). However, with extended follow up (median 17.0 months), remission rates were significantly higher in the rituximab group (64.9 vs. 34.2%, $p < 0.01$).

The Membranous Nephropathy Trial Of Rituximab (MENTOR) study (NCT01180036) was a multicentre, randomised controlled trial comparing the efficacy and safety of rituximab to CsA in medium to high-risk patients with idiopathic MN [78]. Patients with proteinuria ≥5 g/24 hour following a minimum period of 3 months of conservative non-immunosuppressive therapy were randomised to receive IV rituximab 1000 mg (day 1 and 15, then repeated at 6 months) or oral CsA (3.5 mg/kg/day for 12 months). Patients who received CsA had a higher rate of treatment failure at 24 months compared with those who received rituximab (79.4 vs. 37.5%), and CR or PR occurred in 62.5% of the rituximab cohort compared with 20.6% of those who received CsA (odds ratio 6.0, 95% CI 2.7–13.2, $P < 0.0001$).

Numerous prospective uncontrolled studies have been performed evaluating the efficacy of rituximab in idiopathic MN and are summarised in **Table 1** [75, 77–87].

14.6 Eculizumab

Eculizumab is a humanised anti-C5 monoclonal antibody designed to prevent the cleavage of C5 into its proinflammatory by-products. In a randomised placebo-controlled trial in 200 patients with MN, eculizumab, although well-tolerated, failed to show any significant reduction of proteinuria. There were concerns that the dosing schedules were inadequate as inhibition of complement was not uniformly demonstrated. Patients in the eculizumab arm were treated every 2 weeks with two different intravenous dose regimens over a total of 16 weeks [88]. Neither of the active drug regimens of eculizumab showed any significant effect on proteinuria or kidney function compared to placebo. More encouraging results were seen in a continuation of the original study, in which eculizumab was used for up to 1 year, with a significant reduction in proteinuria in some patients (including two patients who went into CR). More long-term studies need to be performed with anti-C5 monoclonal antibody to determine its role in the treatment of MN.

14.7 Adrenocorticotropic hormone

In a study by Berg and colleagues, synthetic adrenocorticotropic hormone (ACTH) administered 1 mg twice per week for 1 year decreased proteinuria in patients with idiopathic MN [89, 90]. Ponticelli et al. conducted a randomised pilot study comparing methylprednisolone plus a cytotoxic agent versus synthetic ACTH in 32 patients with idiopathic MN [91]. In this study, 16 patients were randomly assigned to receive three cycles of MTP (IV MTP 1 g, administered for 3 consecutive days, and then 0.4 mg/kg body weight per day for 27 days, administered orally) and each cycle was followed by 1 month of treatment with either chlorambucil (0.2 mg/kg/day orally) or cyclophosphamide (2.5 mg/kg/day orally), and 16 were assigned to receive ACTH 1 mg intramuscular injections administered initially one injection every other week to two injections per week for a total treatment period of 1 year. No significant differences were observed in remission rates between the ACTH and control groups (87 vs. 93%, respectively), Medication discontinuation rates due to lack of efficacy or adverse drug reactions were 12.5% in both groups. A pilot study by Hladunewich et al. administered 20 idiopathic MN patients with either 40 or 80 IU twice-weekly dose of Acthar® gel and found a significant improvement in proteinuria at 12 months in the entire cohort [92]. There was >50% decrease in proteinuria in 65% of patients and no significant adverse effects were documented. Improvement in serum anti-PLA_2R antibodies was not noted in all patients. Measured anti-PLA2R antibodies became undetectable in three out of 15 patients and appreciably declined in another four patients.

A suggested, risk-based treatment algorithm is displayed in **Figure 4**. It is intended as a guide only and should additionally take into account individual patient circumstances and preferences. Patients who do not respond well or relapse after a first course of immunosuppression therapy may benefit from a second course of immunosuppression.

Patients with severe kidney insufficiency (serum creatinine of ≥3.5 mg/dL or 309 μmol/L) are less likely to benefit from immunosuppression therapy and more likely to experience treatment-related harm, such that consideration should be given to conservative therapy only and plans made for transplantation in the future [41].

Author/year	Level of evidence	Risk group	N	Treatment regimens	Median follow-up (months)	Outcomes/comments
Dahan/2017 [77]	RCT	Medium-high	75	RTX 375 mg/m^2 on day 1 and 8 + NIAT vs. NIAT alone	17	At 6 months, 13 of 37 (35.1%) treated with RTX + NIAT achieved remission vs. 8 of 38 (21.1%) controls (p = 0.21). Significantly higher rates of PLA_2R antibody depletion at 3 and 6 months in RTX + NIAT group.
Fiorentino/2016 [79]	Prospective uncontrolled	Medium-high	38	RTX 375 mg/m^2 monthly × 6	15	29 of 38 (76.3%) achieved remission –15 (39.5%) CR and 14 (36.8%) PR. Proteinuria significantly reduced. Kidney function stable. No significant adverse events.
Bagchi/2018 [80]	Retrospective uncontrolled	High	21	RTX 500 mg × 2 doses 7–10 days apart ± 3rd dose after 4–6 weeks if CD19 not depleted	13	13 of 21 (61.9%) achieved remission –4 (19.05) CR and 9 (42.9%) PR. One patient relapsed after achieving PR. Kidney survival was significantly better in responders (p –0.0037).
Moroni [81]	Prospective uncontrolled	Medium-high	34	RTX 375 mg/m^2 × 1 dose (n = 18) or ×2 2 weeks apart (n = 16)	23.9 (mean)	At 12 months, 5 (14.7%) CR, 10 (29.4%) PR and 19 (55.8%) no response. Outcome similar for one vs. two doses.
Waldman/2016 [82]	Prospective	High	13	CsA 3 mg/kg/day for 6 months then tapered by 50 mg/day every 3 weeks plus RTX 1000 mg day 1 and 15, then after 6 months when CD19+ B cell count ≥5 cells/μL.	41 (mean)	By 6 months 85% achieved remission (CR + PR). By 12 months, 54% achieved CR. 2 relapsed by 24 months. Treatment well tolerated.
Ruggenenti/2015 [83]	Prospective	High	132	RTX 375 mg/m^2 weekly ×4	30.8	84 of 132 (63.6%) achieved remission (CR + PR), 43 (32.6%) achieved CR. Anti-PLA_2R antibody depletion preceded remission.
Ruggenenti/2003 [75]	Prospective	Medium	8	RTX 375 mg/m^2 weekly ×4	Not specified	Significant reduction in proteinuria. Kidney function stabilised. two achieved CR and three achieved PR.

Author/year	Level of evidence	Risk group	N	Treatment regimens	Median follow-up (months)	Outcomes/comments
Ruggenenti/2012 [84]	Prospective	High	100	RTX 375 mg/m^2 weekly ×4	29 (median)	At end of follow up, 65% achieved CR or PR. Median time to remission 7.1 months. Kidney function improved in those who achieved CR.
Fervenza/2010 [85]	Prospective	Medium	20	RTX 375 mg/m^2 weekly ×4, repeated at 6 months	Not specified	Proteinuria reduced from 11.9 g/24 hours to 4.2 and 2.0 g/24 hours at 12 and 24 months, respectively. At 24 months, 4 of 18 achieved CR, 12 of 18 achieved PR and 1 relapsed. Remission rates higher than fortnightly dosing.
Fervenza/2008 [86]	Prospective	High	14	RTX 1000 mg on day 1 and 15, repeated at 6 months if proteinuria >3 g/24 hours and CD9 + B cell >15 cells/μL	12	At 6 months, four achieved PR. At 12 months, two achieved CR and 6 PR.
Fervenza/2015 [78] Results from abstract	RCT	High	130	RTX 1000 mg on day 1 and 15, repeated at 6 months vs. CsA 3.5–5 mg/kg/day for 6 months	24	At 24 months, CR or PR in RTX arm was 62.5 vs. 20.6% in the CsA arm Treatment failure higher in CsA group compared to RTX group (79.4 vs. 37.5%).
Rojas-Rivera/2015 [87]	RCT	High		MTP 1 g IV day 1–3 then MTP PO 0.5 mg/kg/day for day 4–30 on months 1, 3 and 5 and cyclophosphamide PO 2.0 mg/kg/day for 30 days on months 2, 4 and 6 vs. tacrolimus 0.05 mg/kg/day for 6 months, then tapered to withdrawal by 9 months + RTX 1 g at day 180.		Results awaited

Abbreviations are: RCT, randomised controlled trial; RTX, rituximab; NIAT, non-immunosuppressive antiproteinuric therapy; CsA, cyclosporine; CR, CR; PR, partial remission; MTP, methylprednisolone; PO, per oral.

Table 1.
Rituximab treatment of idiopathic MN.

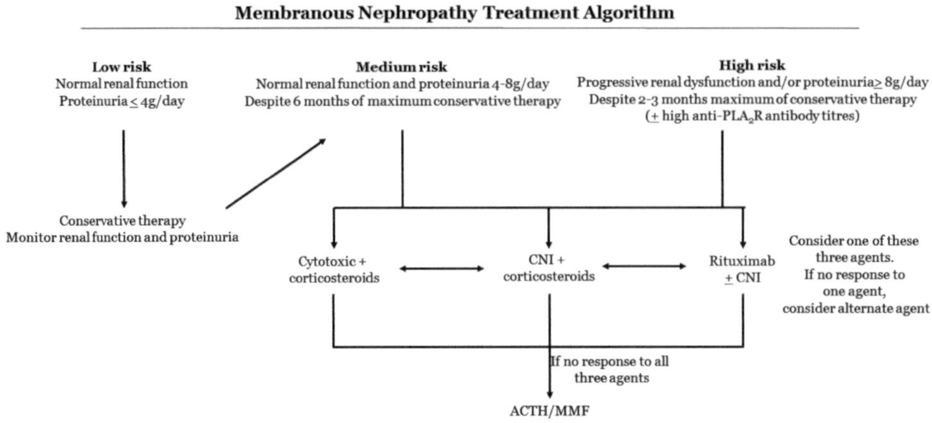

Figure 4.

*Treatment algorithm for idiopathic MN. Based on the renal function and degree of proteinuria at presentation, patients with MN can be classified in to low, medium and high risk category for progression. Patients in the low risk category should be managed with conservative therapy alone but during follow up if they transform in to medium or high risk category then they should be considered for immunosuppressive therapy. Patients in the medium risk category should be treated with conservative therapy for at least 6 months and despite that if they still have more than 4 g/day of proteinuria then they should be considered for immunosuppressive therapy. Patients in the high risk category shouldn't wait for 6 months before starting immunosuppressive therapy. Patients in the medium or high risk category could be treated with either cytotoxics plus corticosteroids or CNI plus corticosteroids or rituximab with or without CNI. If there is no response to one agent, consider alternate agent. If the patient is refractory to all three agents, then they could be treated either with MMF or ACTH. *Conservative treatment involves the use of ACEi ± ARB blocker to maintain BP < 125/75 mmHg, lipid control with HMG-CoA reductase inhibitor, dietary protein restriction (0.6–0.8 g/kg ideal body weight/day), dietary NaCl intake (goal is 2–3 g Na) to optimise antiproteinuric effects of ACEi and ARBs, smoking cessation, and attempt to reduce obesity, if present. Abbreviations are: anti-PLA2R, phospholipase A_2 receptor antibody; ACEi, angiotensin converting enzyme inhibitor; ARB, angiotensin II receptor blocker; CNI, calcineurin inhibitor; ACTH, adrenocorticotrophic hormone; MMF, mycophenolate mofetil.*

15. Conclusion

In conclusion, controlling proteinuria (either CR or PR) in MN is clearly associated with a slower rate of kidney disease progression. Newer biomarkers, such anti-PLA2R antibody and THSD7A, are showing some promising role in differentiating between primary versus secondary MN, predicting prognosis and response to therapy. There are no standard or universal first-line specific therapeutic options for idiopathic MN. Supportive or conservative care, including dietary salt restriction, anti-proteinuric therapy with ACEi or ARB, optimisation of blood pressure and serum cholesterol, and management of cardiovascular and thromboembolic risks, should be given in all cases. Immunosuppressive therapy, such as cytotoxic agents and steroids, calcineurin inhibitors and steroids, rituximab (with or without calcineurin inhibitors), and ACTH, should be considered in patients at medium or high risk of kidney disease progression, cardiovascular disease or thromboembolic complications, as evidenced by heavy proteinuria (>4 g/day) and/or deteriorating kidney function.

Acknowledgements

The authors would like to thank Dr. Jasveen Renthawa for providing the renal biopsy images.

Conflict of interest

Authors declare no conflict of interest.

Author details

Bhadran Bose[1,2], Sunil V. Badve[2,3,4], Vivekanand Jha[5,6,7], Chen Au Peh[8,9] and David Johnson[2,10,11*]

1 Department of Nephrology, Nepean Hospital, Kingswood, Australia

2 Australasian Kidney Trials Network, University of Queensland, Brisbane, Australia

3 Department of Nephrology, St George Hospital, Sydney, Australia

4 The George Institute for Global Health, Sydney, Australia

5 The George Institute for Global Health, New Delhi, India

6 University of Oxford, Oxford, UK

7 University of New South Wales, Sydney, Australia

8 Department of Renal Medicine, Royal Adelaide Hospital, Adelaide, Australia

9 University of Adelaide, Adelaide, Australia

10 Department of Nephrology, Princess Alexandra Hospital, Brisbane, Australia

11 Translational Research Institute, Brisbane, Australia

*Address all correspondence to: david.johnson2@health.qld.gov.au

References

[1] Swaminathan S, Leung N, Lager DJ, Melton LJ 3rd, Bergstralh EJ, Rohlinger A, et al. Changing incidence of glomerular disease in Olmsted County, Minnesota: A 30-year renal biopsy study. Clinical Journal of the American Society of Nephrology. 2006;**1**(3):483-487

[2] Haas M, Meehan SM, Karrison TG, Spargo BH. Changing etiologies of unexplained adult nephrotic syndrome: A comparison of renal biopsy findings from 1976-1979 and 1995-1997. American Journal of Kidney Diseases. 1997;**30**(5):621-631

[3] Glassock RJ. Secondary membranous glomerulonephritis. Nephrology, Dialysis, Transplantation. 1992;**7** (Suppl 1):64-71

[4] Cattran DC, Brenchley PE. Membranous nephropathy: Integrating basic science into improved clinical management. Kidney International. 2017;**91**(3):566-574

[5] Debiec H, Ronco P. Immunopathogenesis of membranous nephropathy: An update. Seminars in Immunopathology. 2014;**36**(4):381-397

[6] De Vriese AS, Glassock RJ, Nath KA, Sethi S, Fervenza FC. A proposal for a serology-based approach to membranous nephropathy. Journal of the American Society of Nephrology. 2017;**28**(2):421-430

[7] Hogan SL, Muller KE, Jennette JC, Falk RJ. A review of therapeutic studies of idiopathic membranous glomerulopathy. American Journal of Kidney Diseases. 1995;**25**(6):862-875

[8] Beck LH, Bonegio RGB, Lambeau G, Beck DM, Powell DW, Cummins TD, et al. M-type phospholipase A_2 receptor as target antigen in idiopathic membranous nephropathy. The New England Journal of Medicine. 2009;**361**(1):11-21

[9] Francis JM, Beck LH Jr, Salant DJ. Membranous nephropathy: A journey from bench to bedside. American Journal of Kidney Diseases. 2016;**68**(1):138-147

[10] Debiec H, Ronco P. Immune response against autoantigen PLA2R is not gambling: Implications for pathophysiology, prognosis, and therapy. Journal of the American Society of Nephrology. 2016;**27**(5):1275-1277

[11] Ronco P, Debiec H. Pathophysiological advances in membranous nephropathy: Time for a shift in patient's care. Lancet. 2015;**385**(9981):1983-1992

[12] Sinico RA, Mezzina N, Trezzi B, Ghiggeri GM, Radice A. Immunology of membranous nephropathy: From animal models to humans. Clinical and Experimental Immunology. 2016;**183**(2):157-165

[13] Hoxha E, Kneissler U, Stege G, Zahner G, Thiele I, Panzer U, et al. Enhanced expression of the M-type phospholipase A2 receptor in glomeruli correlates with serum receptor antibodies in primary membranous nephropathy. Kidney International. 2012;**82**(7):797-804

[14] Larsen CP, Messias NC, Silva FG, Messias E, Walker PD. Determination of primary versus secondary membranous glomerulopathy utilizing phospholipase A_2 receptor staining in renal biopsies. Modern Pathology. 2013;**26**(5):709-715

[15] Xie Q, Li Y, Xue J, Xiong Z, Wang L, Sun Z, et al. Renal phospholipase A2 receptor in hepatitis B virus-associated membranous nephropathy.

American Journal of Nephrology. 2015;**41**(4-5):345-353

[16] Stanescu HC, Arcos-Burgos M, Medlar A, Bockenhauer D, Kottgen A, Dragomirescu L, et al. Risk HLA-DQA1 and PLA(2)R1 alleles in idiopathic membranous nephropathy. The New England Journal of Medicine. 2011;**364**(7):616-626

[17] Lv J, Hou W, Zhou X, Liu G, Zhou F, Zhao N, et al. Interaction between PLA2R1 and HLA-DQA1 variants associates with anti-PLA2R antibodies and membranous nephropathy. Journal of the American Society of Nephrology. 2013;**24**(8):1323-1329

[18] Kanigicherla D, Gummadova J, McKenzie EA, Roberts SA, Harris S, Nikam M, et al. Anti-PLA2R antibodies measured by ELISA predict long-term outcome in a prevalent population of patients with idiopathic membranous nephropathy. Kidney International. 2013;**83**(5):940-948

[19] Ancian P, Lambeau G, Mattei MG, Lazdunski M. The human 180-kDa receptor for secretory phospholipases A_2. Molecular cloning, identification of a secreted soluble form, expression, and chromosomal localization. The Journal of Biological Chemistry. 1995;**270**(15):8963-8970

[20] Fresquet M, Jowitt TA, Gummadova J, Collins R, O'Cualain R, McKenzie EA, et al. Identification of a major epitope recognized by PLA2R autoantibodies in primary membranous nephropathy. Journal of the American Society of Nephrology. 2015;**26**(2):302-313

[21] Seitz-Polski B, Dolla G, Payre C, Girard CA, Polidori J, Zorzi K, et al. Epitope spreading of autoantibody response to PLA2R associates with poor prognosis in membranous nephropathy. Journal of the American Society of Nephrology. 2016;**27**(5):1517-1533

[22] Tomas NM, Beck LH, Meyer-Schwesinger C, Seitz-Polski B, Ma H, Zahner G, et al. Thrombospondin type-1 domain-containing 7A in idiopathic membranous nephropathy. The New England Journal of Medicine. 2014;**371**(24):2277-2287

[23] Ren S, Wu C, Zhang Y, Wang AY, Li G, Wang L, et al. An update on clinical significance of use of THSD7A in diagnosing idiopathic membranous nephropathy: A systematic review and meta-analysis of THSD7A in IMN. Renal Failure. 2018;**40**(1):306-313

[24] Larsen CP, Cossey LN, Beck LH. THSD7A staining of membranous glomerulopathy in clinical practice reveals cases with dual autoantibody positivity. Modern Pathology. 2016;**29**(4):421-426

[25] Gluck MC, Gallo G, Lowenstein J, Baldwin DS. Membranous glomerulonephritis. Evolution of clinical and pathologic features. Annals of Internal Medicine. 1973;**78**(1):1-12

[26] Schieppati A, Mosconi L, Perna A, Mecca G, Bertani T, Garattini S, et al. Prognosis of untreated patients with idiopathic membranous nephropathy. The New England Journal of Medicine. 1993;**329**(2):85-89

[27] Hladunewich MA, Troyanov S, Calafati J, Cattran DC, Metropolitan Toronto Glomerulonephritis Registry. The natural history of the non-nephrotic membranous nephropathy patient. Clinical Journal of the American Society of Nephrology. 2009;**4**(9):1417-1422

[28] Ramzy MH, Cameron JS, Turner DR, Neild GH, Ogg CS, Hicks J. The long-term outcome of idiopathic membranous nephropathy. Clinical Nephrology. 1981;**16**(1):13-19

[29] O'Callaghan CA, Hicks J, Doll H, Sacks SH, Cameron JS. Characteristics

and outcome of membranous nephropathy in older patients. International Urology and Nephrology. 2002;**33**(1):157-165

[30] Lionaki S, Derebail VK, Hogan SL, Barbour S, Lee T, Hladunewich M, et al. Venous thromboembolism in patients with membranous nephropathy. Clinical Journal of the American Society of Nephrology. 2012;7(1):43-51

[31] Donadio JV Jr, Torres VE, Velosa JA, Wagoner RD, Holley KE, Okamura M, et al. Idiopathic membranous nephropathy: The natural history of untreated patients. Kidney International. 1988;**33**(3):708-715

[32] Erwin DT, Donadio JV Jr, Holley KE. The clinical course of idiopathic membranous nephropathy. Mayo Clinic Proceedings. 1973;**48**(10):697-712

[33] Glassock RJ. Diagnosis and natural course of membranous nephropathy. Seminars in Nephrology. 2003;**23**(4):324-332

[34] Timmermans SA, Abdul Hamid MA, Cohen Tervaert JW, Damoiseaux JG, van Paassen P, Limburg Renal Registry. Anti-PLA2R antibodies as a prognostic factor in PLA2R-related membranous nephropathy. American Journal of Nephrology. 2015;**42**(1):70-77

[35] Trew PA, Biava CG, Jacobs RP, Hopper J Jr. Renal vein thrombosis in membranous glomerulonephropathy: Incidence and association. Medicine (Baltimore). 1978;**57**(1):69-82

[36] Wagoner RD, Stanson AW, Holley KE, Winter CS. Renal vein thrombosis in idiopathic membranous glomerulopathy and nephrotic syndrome: Incidence and significance. Kidney International. 1983;**23**(2):368-374

[37] Wehrmann M, Bohle A, Bogenschutz O, Eissele R, Freislederer A, Ohlschlegel C, et al. Long-term prognosis of chronic idiopathic membranous glomerulonephritis. An analysis of 334 cases with particular regard to tubulo-interstitial changes. Clinical Nephrology. 1989;**31**(2):67-76

[38] Pei Y, Cattran D, Greenwood C. Predicting chronic renal insufficiency in idiopathic membranous glomerulonephritis. Kidney International. 1992;**42**(4):960-966

[39] Oh YJ, Yang SH, Kim DK, Kang SW, Kim YS. Autoantibodies against phospholipase A2 receptor in Korean patients with membranous nephropathy. PLoS ONE. 2013;**8**(4):e62151

[40] Hoxha E, Harendza S, Pinnschmidt H, Panzer U, Stahl RA. PLA2R antibody levels and clinical outcome in patients with membranous nephropathy and non-nephrotic range proteinuria under treatment with inhibitors of the renin-angiotensin system. PLoS ONE. 2014;**9**(10):e110681

[41] KDIGO clinical practice guidelines for glomerulonephritis. Kidney International. Supplement. 2012;(S2):139-274

[42] Ponticelli C, Passerini P, Altieri P, Locatelli F, Pappalettera M. Remissions and relapses in idiopathic membranous nephropathy. Nephrology, Dialysis, Transplantation. 1992;7(Suppl 1):85-90

[43] Troyanov S, Wall CA, Miller JA, Scholey JW, Cattran DC, Toronto Glomerulonephritis Registry Group. Idiopathic membranous nephropathy: Definition and relevance of a partial remission. Kidney International. 2004;**66**(3):1199-1205

[44] Ramachandran R, Yadav AK, Kumar V, Inamdar N, Nada R, Gupta KL, et al. Temporal association between PLA2R antibodies and clinical outcomes in primary membranous nephropathy. Kidney International Reports. 2018;**3**(1):142-147

[45] Xie X, Atkins E, Lv J, Bennett A, Neal B, Ninomiya T, et al. Effects of intensive blood pressure lowering on cardiovascular and renal outcomes: Updated systematic review and meta-analysis. Lancet. 2016;**387**(10017):435-443

[46] Peterson JC, Adler S, Burkart JM, Greene T, Hebert LA, Hunsicker LG, et al. Blood pressure control, proteinuria, and the progression of renal disease. The modification of diet in renal disease study. Annals of Internal Medicine. 1995;**123**(10):754-762

[47] Ruggenenti P, Perna A, Gherardi G, Garini G, Zoccali C, Salvadori M, et al. Renoprotective properties of ACE-inhibition in non-diabetic nephropathies with non-nephrotic proteinuria. Lancet. 1999;**354**(9176):359-364

[48] Gansevoort RT, Heeg JE, Vriesendorp R, de Zeeuw D, de Jong PE. Antiproteinuric drugs in patients with idiopathic membranous glomerulopathy. Nephrology, Dialysis, Transplantation. 1992;7(Suppl 1):91-96

[49] Spitalewitz S, Porush JG, Cattran D, Wright N. Treatment of hyperlipidemia in the nephrotic syndrome: The effects of pravastatin therapy. American Journal of Kidney Diseases. 1993;**22**(1):143-150

[50] Sarasin FP, Schifferli JA. Prophylactic oral anticoagulation in nephrotic patients with idiopathic membranous nephropathy. Kidney International. 1994;**45**(2):578-585

[51] Perna A, Schieppati A, Zamora J, Giuliano GA, Braun N, Remuzzi G. Immunosuppressive treatment for idiopathic membranous nephropathy: A systematic review. American Journal of Kidney Diseases. 2004;**44**(3):385-401

[52] Cattran DC, Pei Y, Greenwood CM, Ponticelli C, Passerini P, Honkanen E. Validation of a predictive model of idiopathic membranous nephropathy: Its clinical and research implications. Kidney International. 1997;**51**(3):901-907

[53] Cattran DC, Pei Y, Greenwood C. Predicting progression in membranous glomerulonephritis. Nephrology, Dialysis, Transplantation. 1992;7 (Suppl 1):48-52

[54] A controlled study of short-term prednisone treatment in adults with membranous nephropathy. Collaborative study of the adult idiopathic nephrotic syndrome. The New England Journal of Medicine. 1979;**301**(24):1301-1306

[55] Cattran DC, Delmore T, Roscoe J, Cole E, Cardella C, Charron R, et al. A randomized controlled trial of prednisone in patients with idiopathic membranous nephropathy. The New England Journal of Medicine. 1989;**320**(4):210-215

[56] Ponticelli C, Zucchelli P, Imbasciati E, Cagnoli L, Pozzi C, Passerini P, et al. Controlled trial of methylprednisolone and chlorambucil in idiopathic membranous nephropathy. The New England Journal of Medicine. 1984;**310**(15):946-950

[57] Ponticelli C, Zucchelli P, Passerini P, Cesana B, Locatelli F, Pasquali S, et al. A 10-year follow-up of a randomized study with methylprednisolone and chlorambucil in membranous nephropathy. Kidney International. 1995;**48**(5):1600-1604

[58] Ponticelli C, Zucchelli P, Passerini P, Cesana B. Methylprednisolone plus chlorambucil as compared with methylprednisolone alone for the treatment of idiopathic membranous nephropathy. The Italian Idiopathic Membranous Nephropathy Treatment Study Group. The New England Journal of Medicine. 1992;**327**(9):599-603

[59] Ponticelli C, Altieri P, Scolari F, Passerini P, Roccatello D, Cesana B, et al. A randomized study comparing methylprednisolone plus chlorambucil versus methylprednisolone plus cyclophosphamide in idiopathic membranous nephropathy. Journal of the American Society of Nephrology. 1998;**9**(3):444-450

[60] Jha V, Ganguli A, Saha TK, Kohli HS, Sud K, Gupta KL, et al. A randomized, controlled trial of steroids and cyclophosphamide in adults with nephrotic syndrome caused by idiopathic membranous nephropathy. Journal of the American Society of Nephrology. 2007;**18**(6):1899-1904

[61] Faurschou M, Sorensen IJ, Mellemkjaer L, Loft AG, Thomsen BS, Tvede N, et al. Malignancies in Wegener's granulomatosis: Incidence and relation to cyclophosphamide therapy in a cohort of 293 patients. The Journal of Rheumatology. 2008;**35**(1):100-105

[62] Ambalavanan S, Fauvel JP, Sibley RK, Myers BD. Mechanism of the antiproteinuric effect of cyclosporine in membranous nephropathy. Journal of the American Society of Nephrology. 1996;7(2):290-298

[63] Guasch A, Suranyi M, Newton L, Hall BM, Myers BD. Short-term responsiveness of membranous glomerulopathy to cyclosporine. American Journal of Kidney Diseases. 1992;**20**(5):472-481

[64] Cattran DC, Appel GB, Hebert LA, Hunsicker LG, Pohl MA, Hoy WE, et al. Cyclosporine in patients with steroid-resistant membranous nephropathy: A randomized trial. Kidney International. 2001;**59**(4):1484-1490

[65] Meyrier A, Noel LH, Auriche P, Callard P. Long-term renal tolerance of cyclosporin A treatment in adult idiopathic nephrotic syndrome. Collaborative Group of the Societe de Nephrologie. Kidney International. 1994;**45**(5):1446-1456

[66] Alexopoulos E, Papagianni A, Tsamelashvili M, Leontsini M, Memmos D. Induction and long-term treatment with cyclosporine in membranous nephropathy with the nephrotic syndrome. Nephrology, Dialysis, Transplantation. 2006;**21**(11):3127-3132

[67] Praga M, Barrio V, Juarez GF, Luno J. Grupo Espanol de Estudio de la Nefropatia M. Tacrolimus monotherapy in membranous nephropathy: A randomized controlled trial. Kidney International. 2007;**71**(9):924-930

[68] Cameron JS, Healy MJ, Adu D. The Medical Research Council trial of short-term high-dose alternate day prednisolone in idiopathic membranous nephropathy with nephrotic syndrome in adults. The MRC Glomerulonephritis Working Party. The Quarterly Journal of Medicine. 1990;**74**(274):133-156

[69] Howman A, Chapman TL, Langdon MM, Ferguson C, Adu D, Feehally J, et al. Immunosuppression for progressive membranous nephropathy: A UK randomised controlled trial. Lancet. 2013;**381**(9868):744-751

[70] Cattran DC, Greenwood C, Ritchie S, Bernstein K, Churchill DN, Clark WF, et al. A controlled trial of cyclosporine in patients with progressive membranous nephropathy. Canadian Glomerulonephritis Study Group. Kidney International. 1995;**47**(4):1130-1135

[71] Miller G, Zimmerman R 3rd, Radhakrishnan J, Appel G. Use of mycophenolate mofetil in resistant membranous nephropathy. American Journal of Kidney Diseases. 2000;**36**(2):250-256

[72] Choi MJ, Eustace JA, Gimenez LF, Atta MG, Scheel PJ, Sothinathan R,

et al. Mycophenolate mofetil treatment for primary glomerular diseases. Kidney International. 2002;**61**(3):1098-1114

[73] Branten AJ, du Buf-Vereijken PW, Vervloet M, Wetzels JF. Mycophenolate mofetil in idiopathic membranous nephropathy: A clinical trial with comparison to a historic control group treated with cyclophosphamide. American Journal of Kidney Diseases. 2007;**50**(2):248-256

[74] Remuzzi G, Chiurchiu C, Abbate M, Brusegan V, Bontempelli M, Ruggenenti P. Rituximab for idiopathic membranous nephropathy. Lancet. 2002;**360**(9337):923-924

[75] Ruggenenti P, Chiurchiu C, Brusegan V, Abbate M, Perna A, Filippi C, et al. Rituximab in idiopathic membranous nephropathy: A one-year prospective study. Journal of the American Society of Nephrology. 2003;**14**(7):1851-1857

[76] Fervenza FC, Cossio FG, Leung N, Wasiluk A, Cohen I, Wochos D, et al. A pilot study on the use of rituximab for the treatment of idiopathic membranous nephropathy: Preliminary results. Journal of the American Society of Nephrology. 2005;(16):555A

[77] Dahan K, Debiec H, Plaisier E, Cachanado M, Rousseau A, Wakselman L, et al. Rituximab for severe membranous nephropathy: A 6-month trial with extended follow-up. Journal of the American Society of Nephrology. 2017;**28**(1):348

[78] Fervenza FC, Canetta PA, Barbour SJ, Lafayette RA, Rovin BH, Aslam N, et al. A multicenter randomized controlled trial of rituximab versus cyclosporine in the treatment of idiopathic membranous nephropathy (MENTOR). Nephron. 2015;**130**(3):159-168

[79] Fiorentino M, Tondolo F, Bruno F, Infante B, Grandaliano G, Gesualdo L, et al. Treatment with rituximab in idiopathic membranous nephropathy. Clinical Kidney Journal. 2016;**9**(6):788-793

[80] Bagchi S, Subbiah AK, Bhowmik D, Mahajan S, Yadav RK, Kalaivani M, et al. Low-dose rituximab therapy in resistant idiopathic membranous nephropathy: Single-center experience. Clinical Kidney Journal. 2018;**11**(3):337-341

[81] Moroni G, Depetri F, Del Vecchio L, Gallelli B, Raffiotta F, Giglio E, et al. Low-dose rituximab is poorly effective in patients with primary membranous nephropathy. Nephrology, Dialysis, Transplantation. 2017;**32**(10):1691-1696

[82] Waldman M, Beck LH, Braun M, Wilkins K, Balow JE, Austin HA. Membranous nephropathy: Pilot study of a novel regimen combining cyclosporine and rituximab. Kidney International Reports. 2016;**1**(2):73-84

[83] Ruggenenti P, Debiec H, Ruggiero B, Chianca A, Pellé T, Gaspari F, et al. Anti-phospholipase A_2 receptor antibody titer predicts post-rituximab outcome of membranous nephropathy. Journal of the American Society of Nephrology. 2015;**26**(10):2545

[84] Ruggenenti P, Cravedi P, Chianca A, Perna A, Ruggiero B, Gaspari F, et al. Rituximab in idiopathic membranous nephropathy. Journal of the American Society of Nephrology. 2012;**23**(8):1416

[85] Fervenza FC, Abraham RS, Erickson SB, Irazabal MV, Eirin A, Specks U, et al. Rituximab therapy in idiopathic membranous nephropathy: A 2-year study. Clinical Journal of the American Society of Nephrology. 2010;**5**(12):2188

[86] Fervenza FC, Cosio FG, Erickson SB, Specks U, Herzenberg AM, Dillon JJ, et al. Rituximab treatment of idiopathic membranous nephropathy. Kidney International. 2008;**73**(1):117-125

[87] Rojas-Rivera J, Fernandez-Juarez G, Ortiz A, Hofstra J, Gesualdo L, Tesar V, et al. A European multicentre and open-label controlled randomized trial to evaluate the efficacy of Sequential treatment with TAcrolimus-Rituximab versus steroids plus cyclophosphamide in patients with primary MEmbranous Nephropathy: The STARMEN study. Clinical Kidney Journal. 2015;**8**(5):503-510

[88] Appel G, Nachman P, Hogan S, Radhakrishnan J, Old C, Hebert L, et al. Eculizumab (C5 complement inhibitor) in the treatment of idiopathic membranous nephropathy (abstract). Journal of the American Society of Nephrology. 2002;(13):668A

[89] Berg AL, Nilsson-Ehle P, Arnadottir M. Beneficial effects of ACTH on the serum lipoprotein profile and glomerular function in patients with membranous nephropathy. Kidney International. 1999;**56**(4):1534-1543

[90] Berg AL, Arnadottir M. ACTH-induced improvement in the nephrotic syndrome in patients with a variety of diagnoses. Nephrology, Dialysis, Transplantation. 2004;**19**(5):1305-1307

[91] Ponticelli C, Passerini P, Salvadori M, Manno C, Viola BF, Pasquali S, et al. A randomized pilot trial comparing methylprednisolone plus a cytotoxic agent versus synthetic adrenocorticotropic hormone in idiopathic membranous nephropathy. American Journal of Kidney Diseases. 2006;**47**(2):233-240

[92] Hladunewich MA, Cattran D, Beck LH, Odutayo A, Sethi S, Ayalon R, et al. A pilot study to determine the dose and effectiveness of adrenocorticotrophic hormone (H.P. Acthar(R) Gel) in nephrotic syndrome due to idiopathic membranous nephropathy. Nephrology, Dialysis, Transplantation. 2014;**29**(8):1570-1577

Chapter 5

Primary Membranous Nephropathy as a Model of Autoimmune Disease

Patrick Hamilton, Durga Kanigicherla and Paul Brenchley

Abstract

Membranous nephropathy is the most common cause of adult nephrotic syndrome worldwide with a significant health care burden. There has been a leap in our understanding of the disease mechanism over the last decade with a remarkably strong genetic component to the development of the disease and its strong association with high affinity antibody—in the form of anti-PLA2R autoantibody in the majority of cases, with a smaller proportion associated with anti-THSD7A autoantibody. New evidence is now providing confirmation of specific elements in the development of the disease pathogenesis, such as involvement of loss of peripheral tolerance. There is a striking correlation between disease activity and anti-PLA2R antibody levels, along with response to treatment; evidence points strongly to these antibodies being pathogenic. The development of membranous nephropathy therefore follows the well appreciated multi-hit step-wise path to autoimmune clinical disease. Given its strong genetic basis and putative pathogenic antibody the disease provides an invaluable model for understanding of autoimmunity. This chapter focuses on the most up to date knowledge of autoimmune membranous nephropathy and provides a paradigm for understanding the underlying disease mechanisms in autoimmunity.

Keywords: autoimmune disease, membranous nephropathy, nephrotic syndrome, anti-PLA_2R

1. Introduction

Autoimmune disease is a term that covers a range of conditions in which the immune system recognises the body as a foreign pathogen, and encompasses over 80 conditions affecting almost every organ [1]. Individually, many of these conditions are rare but taken together they represent a significant mortality and morbidity affecting approximately 9% of the population worldwide with the prevalence rising [1, 2]. Given that the majority of conditions have no cure and potentially require lifelong treatment, and that most patients are diagnosed during young adulthood or in middle age, the cost to healthcare systems is particularly significant.

Despite the variation of organs affected and clinical presentation, many of the conditions that appear distinct will share a common theme of disease pathogenesis. Underscoring many of the conditions is a genetic susceptibility that taken in concert with an environmental trigger sets off an immune cascade resulting in the end organ damage and clinical signs and symptoms that bring the patient to the attention of their healthcare provider, the so-called multi-hit hypothesis. As science progresses and we gain greater insight into these disease processes, it is becoming more apparent that there are similarities in many of the conditions. At present, most management strategies attempt to globally restrict the immune system, a strategy that has been shown to help control the disease but comes with a significant side effect profile. Despite the accelerating knowledge we are gaining of the underlying pathogenesis, there remains a lack of directed novel therapies for patients at present, although in many conditions there are signs that this is changing.

Membranous nephropathy represents a particularly interesting basis to understand this process given its clear pathological classification, strong genetic contribution, putative pathogenic antibody and evidence for the loss of tolerance that is now emerging. In this chapter, we review the current understanding of autoimmune membranous nephropathy and use it as a basis for the understanding of autoimmune disease in general.

2. Background

Membranous nephropathy (MN) is the most common cause of nephrotic syndrome in adults worldwide but despite this remains a rare disease. Incidence is estimated at 1.2 per 100,000 in European cohorts with a peak incidence in the fifth and sixth decades, although it can affect any age, and has a slight male preponderance [3]. The classical presentation of the disease is with nephrotic syndrome, that is, the tetrad of leg swelling, proteinuria and serum hypoalbuminemia, with or without hypercholesterolemia. A number of patients have also been known to present with venous thrombosis. This can be in the form of deep vein thrombosis (DVT) and, not uncommonly as the first presentation of the disease, with acute kidney injury (AKI) as a result of renal vein thrombosis. Hypercoagulopathy as a result of the loss of anti-thrombotic factors such as anti-thrombin III and plasminogen due to proteinuria, an increased level of factor VIII and fibrinogen, along with an increased platelet hyperaggregability has been noted in nephrotic syndrome whatever the cause. However, compared to other conditions that have a similar degree of proteinuria, MN has a relatively higher risk of venous thrombosis and its associated risks; the mechanism for this association has not been ascertained [4–6].

Clinically there are two distinct forms of MN, but these can be histologically very similar and difficult to differentiate. Both require very different treatment strategies and therefore distinguishing them is imperative. Primary MN accounts for the majority of patients (approximately 75–80%) and has now been shown to be an autoimmune disease. Secondary MN is caused by a multitude of causes including medications, systemic disorders and toxins, and its treatment is therefore aimed at the underlying trigger or condition [7].

It is one of the idiosyncrasies of MN that up to a third of patients if left untreated will achieve spontaneous remission within the first 2 years following diagnosis, and this potential for spontaneous remission has informed the current treatment options, especially for those patients without rapidly progressive renal decline [8]. The mainstay of treatment at present has a focus on the reduction of proteinuria with the use of an renin-angiotensin pathway blockade or immunosuppression if this fails [7]. It has also meant that for many studies, patients undergo three to 6 months of supportive care before they are eligible, in case any response to treatment seen is actually as a result of spontaneous remission. However, with the increasing use, understanding and monitoring of biomarkers such as anti-PLA_2R, treatments are likely to be less empiric in the future.

If patients do reach ESRD and receive a renal transplant, it has been well demonstrated that this can provide a dramatic improvement to not only life expectancy but also quality of life [9–11]. However, this comes with the risk of recurrence of MN following transplantation (up to 34% of patients) despite the judicial use of immunosuppression and can lead to the loss of the graft in up to 50% of these cases. There is some evidence to suggest that receiving a transplant from a living related donor increases the risk of recurrence, but this is far outweighed by the complications associated with remaining on dialysis [12]. Current practice therefore, is to attempt to match HLA antigens as closely as possible to reduce the reliance on immunosuppression to minimise rejection.

For many patients, MN remains a relapsing and remitting disease, requiring lifelong follow up under the care of specialists in tertiary care. Despite being a rare condition, its chronicity, current standard treatments and their associated side-effects, the risk of ESRD, and disease recurrence means it is a disease that has a significant impact on both a patient's quality of life and a healthcare system with finite resources.

3. Diagnosis

Recent advances in biomarker research for MN have shown promising results but at present diagnosis requires biopsy confirmation. Histologically the disease is characterised by thickening of the glomerular basement membrane and spikes seen on silver stain. Immunofluorescence almost universally shows coarse granular immunoglobulin IgG and complement C3 deposition on the capillary wall. Electron microscopy (EM) will show sub-epithelial immune complex deposition (**Figure 1**). It has become apparent over the years that the dominant IgG subclass found histologically (and for antibodies to PLA2R as described below) in primary MN is IgG4 [13–15]. This appears to differ from secondary MN where IgG1 predominates [16]. IgG makes up a significant proportion of serum protein in humans contributing approximately 10–20% of circulating proteins. It can be further subdivided into four subclasses with differing effects. IgG4 is the least abundant of these subclasses and is generally found in response to allergens or in response to repeated exposure to an antigen [17].

New research findings suggest that there may be a class switch involved in primary membranous nephropathy. Here it has been shown that in early MN (stage I of the Ehrenreich and Churg scale) the predominant subclass of antibody is IgG1 but as the disease progresses this changes so that IgG4 predominates [16].

4. Treatment

In primary MN, disease activity is still measured by proteinuria level and renal excretory function despite the advances in anti-PLA$_2$R research. Proteinuria level has been shown to be not only a marker for remission when it is low but also predicts progression to ESRD when increased. If proteinuria reduces through either spontaneous remission or with treatment, then the risk of CKD progression also falls. It is for this reason that the main focus of treatment in primary MN is concerned with control of proteinuria, with or without the use of immunosuppression, generally in the form of the Ponticelli regime (or calcineurin inhibitors if cyclophosphamide is not tolerated or is contraindicated). This regime of rotating high dose intravenous steroids and immunosuppression was first described in the mid-1980s and has been the recommended regime since [7, 18–20]. Despite its success in treating the condition, the Ponticelli regime comes with a significant side effect burden, including an increased risk of infection, osteoporosis, diabetes mellitus, weight gain,

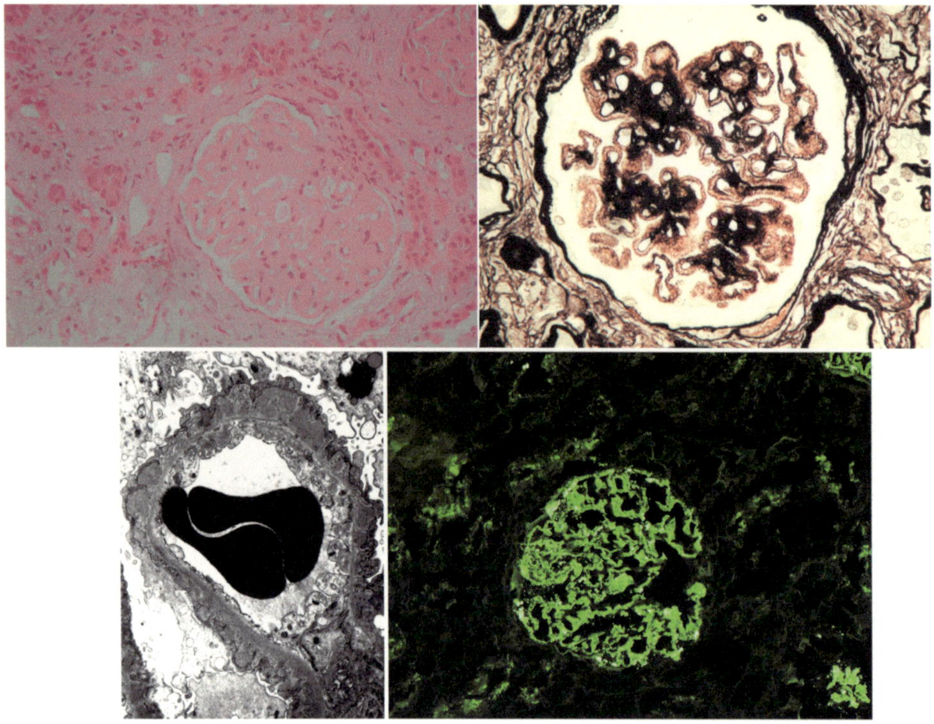

Figure 1.
Histological appearance of membranous nephropathy (a) haematoxylin and eosin stain (H&E) showing marked capillary loop thickening (b) silver staining showing spikes (c) electron microscopy of MN showing sub-epithelial immune complex deposition (d) immunofluorescence showing IgG deposition on the capillary wall. Figures courtesy of Dr. Lorna Williams, Consultant Histopathologist, Manchester University Hospitals Foundation Trust, UK.

haemorrhagic cystitis, infertility and malignancy [18]. It is this that has led many researchers to search for an alternative therapy including mycophenolate mofetil and tacrolimus but with variable evidence to show an improvement in outcomes.

Rituximab is a monoclonal antibody against CD20, found on the B-cells, which leads to a reduction in B-cell numbers and has been used extensively in cancer therapy and autoimmune diseases since its introduction in the 1990s. A number of case series and studies have shown the potential that Rituximab can have for primary MN, but so far there has only been one randomised controlled trial (RCT) [21–24]. Here it has been shown that compared to standard anti-proteinuric therapy, patients treated with rituximab show a greater reduction in anti-PLA_2R levels at month 3, followed by a later reduction in proteinuria, increase in serum albumin and are more likely to enter remission [24]. Combined with the high cost of the medication itself, its widespread use has been restricted in resource-limited, evidence-based healthcare systems, such as the NHS in UK [25]. The use of Rituximab therapy is currently under investigation in the MENTOR study in North America and via the Commissioning through Evaluation pathway run under the auspices of the National Institute for Health and Care Excellence (NICE) in the UK. It is possible that based on these two studies the use of Rituximab will become more ubiquitous in the near future.

5. Future novel treatments

The use of many of these medications comes with side effects that can be unpalatable to the patient and physician and the search for treatments with a reduced side-effect profile is on-going. Treatments such as immunoadsorption (IA) allow for the controlled removal of antibodies without the side effects associated with immunosuppression. Immunoadsorption RCTs in MN though, are non-existent and certainly not in the anti-PLA$_2$R era. Immunoadsorption is a method of removing specific circulating immunoglobulins from the blood and has been shown to remove over 80% of circulating IgG with a single session adsorption of 2.5 plasma volumes, with albumin and antithrombin III almost unaffected [26]. With multiple sessions, this can rise to over 98% [27]. These are removed in the absorber through binding Peptide-GAM. Using two columns per machine, one regenerating whilst the other is removing antibodies; the process can occur indefinitely until the required level of antibody has been removed.

Post IA it appears that autoantibodies can be slow to re-emerge. Use in dilated cardiomyopathy for the removal of β_1-adreno-receptor autoantibodies (β_1-AAB) has shown that only a small minority of patients (0% in the first year and 15% by 3 years) will show an increase in significant β_1-AAB autoantibodies [28, 29].

To our knowledge, there has only been one publication using immunoadsorption for the treatment of MN [30]. In 1999, Esnault et al. successfully used IA for the treatment of various aetiologies of Nephrotic syndrome including four patients with MN [31]. Here they showed that not only is the procedure safe but that there was a significant improvement in proteinuria in all patients with membranous nephropathy. The main side effect in this group of patients was headache, which resolved without sequelae. Since that time the treatment has been used in numerous other autoimmune conditions including Focal Segmental Glomerulosclerosis (FSGS) [32], systemic lupus nephritis (SLE) [33, 34], ANCA-associated small vessel vasculitides [35, 36], Anti-glomerular basement membrane antibody disease [37] and in renal transplantation [38–40].

In conditions such as SLE, the use of immunoadsorption can dramatically reduce the level of circulating immune complexes and autoantibodies leading to clinical improvement in even severe life-threatening SLE. These results have been shown with as little as two sessions within 3 days and repeated every 3 weeks if patients remain with active disease [33]. With the current understanding of primary MN's autoimmune process, the use of IA could provide the ability to rapidly remove the pathogenic antibodies leading to remission. Current IA machines can remove the different classes such as IgG4 with an increased specificity but cannot differentiate further than that. If IA is proved to work for primary MN, it may be possible to develop an IA column that is specific only for anti-PLA$_2$R, therefore allowing for an even more targeted and personalised treatment.

6. Autoimmune membranous nephropathy

Until recently autoimmune (or primary) MN was known as idiopathic MN as its cause remained unclear. It was generally a diagnosis of exclusion, once a patient had biopsy confirmation of MN and all causes of secondary MN had been ruled out. It was for a long time postulated to be an autoimmune disease, but the target antigen in humans remained elusive. In the late 1970s, work on the Heymann Nephritis rat model of experimental MN showed that circulating IgG antibodies could bind to the podocytes [41–43]. The target antigen was found to be megalin, but this was not present on human podocytes, so the search for the target antigen continued. It was not until 2009, almost 40 years later that this was discovered. Here Beck et al. used western blotting with MN patient sera, to show that antibodies bound to a 185 kDa protein band from glomerular extracts. This band was only seen in the primary MN group and not seen in normal patients or other proteinuric conditions including patients with secondary MN. Using mass spectrometry this band was found to contain the M-type phospholipase A2 receptor 1 (PLA2R) [15]. Since then, the increased interest and research into MN has led to the discovery of a second minor target antigen in thrombospondin type-1 domain containing 7A (THSD7A) [44].

7. M-type phospholipase A2 receptor 1

The landmark paper by Beck et al. describing the discovery of autoantibodies to PLA2R found on human podocytes transformed our understanding of the MN disease process. Here was evidence that for the majority of patients with MN, the condition was, as had been postulated, an autoimmune disease [15].

PLA2R is a transmembrane receptor for Phospholipase A2, a protein from the mannose receptor family, one of four described in humans; Endo180, DEC205, Mannose Receptor (MR) and PLA2R [45–47]. As with all the mannose receptor family, the transmembrane glycoprotein has an extracellular component, in the case of PLA2R, this is made up of an N-terminal ricin rich domain, a fibronectin type II domain and 8 C-type lectin domains (CTLDs) [48]. In the kidney, it is found almost exclusively on the podocytes, but it has also been found on neutrophils and in the lung [49, 50]. Its function in the kidney remains unknown, however, and how the anti-PLA_2R antibodies alter its normal function leading to proteinuria, if indeed that is what is part of the process, also remains unknown [15, 51].

The predominant antibody to PLA2R is IgG and in particular IgG4, which is the major component of immune complex deposition in primary MN [13, 14]. These immune complexes appear to form in the kidney with the IgG4 antibodies and the PLA2R antigen being co-localised, giving further evidence for the role of PLA2R in the disease process [52, 53]. The fact that the complexes form in situ in the kidney may explain why some patients with biopsy-proven MN and clinical evidence for the disease are serum anti-PLA_2R negative. Debiec and Ronco showed in 2011 that there were a number of patients who were serum anti-PLA_2R negative but had detectable PLA2R in glomerular deposits. They did also find a few patients with no PLA2R in the glomerular deposits but who were serologically positive [54]. We know that anti-PLA_2R antibodies have a high affinity for PLA2R in the podocytes and it may be that a certain level of deposition is required to overload the system before the anti-PLA_2R antibodies become serologically detectable [48].

Much of the excitement surrounding anti-PLA_2R is due to its apparent pathogenicity with the resultant potential for use as a biomarker and as a treatment target. Several studies have provided evidence for its pathogenicity showing that a high titre correlates with disease activity. For patients who go into remission either spontaneously or through the use of immunosuppression, the anti-PLA_2R level falls months before this becomes clinically apparent with a fall in proteinuria. If a patient relapses, this again is predated by a rise in antibody titres [55–60].

Outcomes can also be predicted with high titres predicting a worse outcome in regards to renal function and an improved outcome with low titres [55]. If treatment does not result in antibody negativity, then they are left with a high risk of relapse [51, 57]. Ruggenenti et al. have shown similar results with a reduction in anti-PLA_2R levels strongly predicting remission and increasing titres following this, predicting relapse [59].

With the increasingly strong evidence for the involvement of anti-PLA_2R antibodies in the pathogenesis of primary MN, the focus has now shifted to trying to understand the antigen and its interaction with the autoantibody. Work carried out in Manchester has now determined the major epitope on the PLA2R antigen that is recognised by the anti-PLA$_2$R antibodies. Four different sized fragments of extracellular PLA2R (full-length N-C8, N-terminus to C-type lectin domain (CTLD) 3 (N-C3), N-terminus to CTLD2 (N-C2) and a ricin rich domain) were used to investigate the reactivity of human anti-PLA$_2$R autoantibodies. It was found that the major epitope was located in the N-C3 region of the receptor. The antibodies were also found to bind with an equal affinity to the four different fragments, confirming the existence of a single epitope. The epitope itself is a 31-mer peptide made up of the beta-1 and beta-3 strands and encompassing the beta-2 strand [48].

Leading on from this the Manchester team also constructed a 3D model of the structure of the immune complex incorporating the extracellular N-C8 PLA2R and the autoantibody with the binding site [48]. This work has been further confirmed by Kao et al. who found that the dominant epitope is in the N-terminal region as well, in particular in the region from the ricin rich domain through the fibronectin-like type to the CTLD1 [61].

8. Thrombospondin type-1 domain-containing 7A

The fact that anti-PLA$_2$R antibodies are found in up to 80% of patients with primary MN raises a number of possibilities. It is known that some patients with secondary membranous can develop malignancies years after the diagnosis of MN and it may be that these patients fall into this category. Whether these patients represent a cohort who have two separate conditions and it is coincidental that one is known to cause the other is still up for debate. A second possibility is that there are more pathogenic antigens leading to the formation of autoantibodies than previously thought. In fact, for a small number of patients with primary MN, this seems to be the case.

Using western blotting, Thomas et al. discovered a glomerular protein of 250 kDa in patients with anti-PLA$_2$R negative biopsy-proven membranous nephropathy. This corresponded to THSD7A, a protein found in the podocyte foot processes [44].

They went on to show that the predominant antibody to this antigen was IgG4 in keeping with a diagnosis of primary MN, and on histological staining, in a similar fashion to anti-PLA$_2$R, the immune complexes were co-localised with the antigen. Levels of the antibody were shown to correlate with disease activity, being higher in active disease and lower as the clinical manifestations of the disease improved. Interestingly, there appeared to be no statistical significance in the clinical presentation or demographics between the anti-PLA$_2$R positive and the anti-THSD7A positive patients, except for a slightly higher number of women in the anti-THSD7A group, although this is believed to be due to the small numbers involved.

This evidence suggests that for a minority of primary MN patients, approximately 2.5–5% in this study, a second unrelated and discrete antigen is involved with the pathogenesis of the disease [44]. Whether this all represents a separate disease and whether there are other minor antigens still to be discovered remains unknown as does the major epitope in THSD7A. However, for PLA2R, in addition to the major epitope in the CysR domain, evidence from the work of Fresquet et al. on the identification of the major epitope of PLA2R, showed that 10% of anti-PLA$_2$R positive sera reacted with an epitope at CTLD4-8. This suggests that there may be a further, as yet unidentified, antibody to this minor epitope [48]. This idea of epitope spreading has been suggested by Lambeau et al. who have defined additional epitopes in CTLD1 and CTLD7 domains [62].

9. The multi-hit hypothesis

9.1 Genetic association

Why some patients develop an autoantibody to PLA2R is still an unknown, but it does appear to have a strong genetic component. The first clue to the genetic basis of the disease was the discovery of the association with Human Leucocyte Antigen (HLA)—DR3 followed closely by the identification of familial clustering in 1984 [30, 63, 64]. Following the discovery of the PLA2R antigen, researchers studying Korean and Chinese populations investigated the association of a number of single nucleotide polymorphisms (SNPs) known to be associated with PLA2R. They both found that a polymorphism at rs35771982 was significantly associated with primary MN. Interestingly, this polymorphism is located on CTLD1, in the region that was later found to contain an epitope in the antigen [48, 65, 66].

The major Genome-Wide Association Study (GWAS) in MN of 556 patients (French, Dutch and British) revealed two major loci of allelic association. The first is not unexpectedly on chromosome 6p21 within HLA-DQA1 gene, and the second is on chromosome 2q24 containing PLA2R1. For patients who were homozygous for these alleles, their odds ratio for having primary membranous nephropathy was 78.5 [67]. This work has recently been validated in a study using genotype and HLA imputation alongside a GWAS in 323 patients with primary MN. Here the association of HLA-DQA1 and PLA2R1 with primary MN was confirmed, without detecting any other novel signals [68].

How these genetic markers modulate the risk of developing MN is unknown. The idea that the genetically restricted class II presentation of PLA2R peptides to affect the class switch to high-affinity IgG anti-PLA_2R is a theory that remains to be tested.

9.2 Environmental trigger

Indicative of the rapid pace of research into primary MN since the discovery of the PLA2R antigen, we now have not only the clinical correlation of the antibody with disease activity but also the major epitope on the antigen and evidence for the genetic polymorphism located in the antigen itself. This, however, does not completely explain the development of the disease. The polymorphisms described in these studies are actually variants that are common to the general population. It seems likely that, similar to other autoimmune diseases such as IgA nephropathy, primary MN is a multi-hit disease. A patient with the polymorphism has a genetic predisposition but to develop the disease needs an external trigger.

Fresquet et al. have shown that an amino acid sequence which is part of the dominant epitope in the CysR region of the PLA_2R antigen is also found in the cell wall of some species of clostridia [48]. Further searches using the Basic Local Alignment Search Tool (BLAST) [69] has shown this peptide sequence is found in a number of other common pathogens such as Pseudomonas and *Saccharomyces cerevisiae*.

There is now also emerging evidence implicating air pollution in the development of autoimmune MN. A recent large study in China investigating the emerging trends of glomerulopathy based on renal biopsies in relation to air pollution noted a rise in the incidence of MN in all age ranges and in all regions, this is in contrast to other glomerular disease investigated which all remained the same. It was more prevalent in areas with the highest air pollution and the long-term average was found to be associated with a significantly increased risk of autoimmune MN.

9.3 Loss of tolerance

What is not known at present is the risk of developing autoimmune MN if you have the genetic predisposition, only that you are more likely to have the risk alleles if you have autoimmune MN. What remains elusive is how a patient's immune system converts from an advantageous defence against common pathogens to a pathogenic entity in itself. A characteristic of autoimmune MN is the heterogeneity shown in prognosis and its waxing and waning nature over time. A proportion of patients will undergo a phenomenon of spontaneous remission, and in patients with a more severe phenotype, it is not unusual for them to follow a relapsing and remitting course. Many patients, when they first come to medical attention, will describe self-limiting episodes many months or years prior to their diagnosis that is likely to be nephrotic states and the first signs of the disease. This suggests that far from being a continuously progressive immunological process, particularly in light of the pathogenicity of the autoantibody, that there may be natural mechanisms at play attempting to maintain a balance. Work in other autoimmune diseases such as autoimmune thyroiditis has proven the existence of antigens capable of maintaining a population of natural T Regs and thereby keeping pathogenic antibodies suppressed [70].

As the technology evolves, flow cytometry is becoming an ever more powerful tool for the study of the immune system. A recent study using patients enrolled in the GEMRITUX trial showed that patients had lower proportions of IgD− and IgD+ memory B cells, T Regs and a higher proportion of naïve B cells at baseline compared to healthy donors [71]. In this study by Rosenzwajg et al., patients who responded to treatment were observed to have a lower proportion of T Regs at baseline compared to those who did not respond to treatment. They also noted that in patients with no response to treatment, there was no increase in T Regs following treatment, however in patients who went on to respond, there was a significantly higher proportion of T Regs at day 8 compared to baseline [71].

This is similar to work currently being undertaken in our lab (unpublished) in which flow cytometry was used to model the immune system following treatment with immunoadsorption [72]. In our cohort, we also found that there was a lower proportion of IgD+ memory B cells in the patient group but a similar level of IgD− memory B cells albeit with a much larger range. For the Naïve B cells and T Regs, the medians were very similar between the patients and control group but with a much larger range in the patient cohort. One of the striking differences between our patient group and the control group at baseline is that there does not seem to be any statistical difference in PLA_2R positive B cells, with a number of volunteers in the control group showing a relatively high proportion of these cells. This seemingly counterintuitive result, in fact, appears to add weight to the importance of loss of tolerance in the disease process.

Given the shared sequence of amino acids (SVLTLENC), it could be expected during the development of normal natural immunity to a range of pathogens, developing IgM antibodies to this linear peptide sequence is common, entirely normal and beneficial to the host. The risk of developing an autoimmune pathology only arises then, if a patient has the genetic makeup (pathological alleles of DQA1 and PLA2R) required to present PLA_2R T cell peptides to their immune system. Only with the permissive genetic background and continued exposure to the pathogen or environmental trigger, causing immune processing of PLA_2R, will class switching occur from IgM to IgG, and therefore allowing the development of pathogenic high-affinity antibodies. In our PLA_2R panel, the healthy control group showed a significant level of PLA_2R positive B cells. A current on-going and unpublished project being carried out in our lab is the development of an IgM anti-PLA_2R

ELISA. Although it cannot be proven in the current flow cytometry experiment, it would appear to suggest that there is a high likelihood that the B cells seen in the healthy population may, in fact, be IgM positive B cells as opposed to being IgG positive.

A further interesting dimension to immune regulation and loss of tolerance that needs further study is the role that T reg cells play and how they are a potential mechanism for the suppression of pathogenic antibodies. The relapsing and remitting nature of autoimmune membranous nephropathy and the phenomenon of spontaneous remission indicates that at some level there must be an immune mechanism capable of suppressing the anti-PLA_2R antibodies, much like that found in autoimmune thyroiditis. Another on-going study, again unpublished, in our lab has identified a number of healthy controls without the prerequisite HLA-DQA1 or PLA2R1 genes needed to develop autoimmune MN, who have a detectable level of circulating soluble PLA_2R using mouse anti-PLA_2R as the capture antibody. There is the potential that these circulating soluble-PLA_2R antigens are active in maintaining a functioning level of T Regs to suppress class switching and downregulate the pathogenic antibody level. If natural T Regs did indeed have a role in keeping the pathogenic IgG anti-PLA_2R antibodies suppressed, the expectation would be that in times of active disease the levels would be low. The opposite would also be true with high levels in times of remission or just before remission or response to treatment. The T cell panel used for the patient cohort does start to show a pattern of T Regs change over time, a pattern that appears to support the theory above, especially when taken in the context of antibody level. At week 4 follow up, the T Regs level has dropped to their lowest point, this is also at the same time point at which the anti-PLA_2R is at its highest. The proportion of T Regs then show an increase at both week 10 and week 16 follow up, just as the antibody level is decreasing.

10. Summary

Autoimmune MN has experienced a step change in our understanding of the disease pathogenesis since the discovery of the anti-PLA_2R autoantibody in 2009 [15], however, there is much that still remains unknown. Despite the advances seen over the last decade, the management of the disease remains an empirical treatment based on a regimen first introduced over two decades ago. There is as yet no disease-specific therapy or alternative to glucocorticoids and immunosuppression in mainstream use.

As with all autoimmune diseases, the eventual clinically apparent symptoms are the end result in a journey of multiple steps, the so-called multi-hit hypothesis. We know that there is a strong genetic component in the development of the disease, with patients homozygous for both the HLA-DQA1 and PLA2R1 genes are almost 80 times more likely to develop the disease than patients who do not [67]. What we still do not know is whether the possession of these genes in itself guarantees the development of the disease. It is likely that a further trigger (likely environmental) is required to progress to the disease state.

Development of the normal natural immunity requires the production of antibodies, including IgM, to linear peptides in a whole range of epitopes. With this beneficial protective immunity, circulating IgM antibodies to the PLA_2R p28mer peptide can, in fact, be a normal occurrence. The presence of these antibodies in patients without the genetic predisposition to the disease would just be an expected variant of normal. It is in those patients who do have the genetic predisposition to developing the disease, that the presence of IgM antibodies with the ability to recognise the p28mer will have the potential to progress to the disease state to generate a high-affinity IgG response. Once this occurs, and there is recognition of the podocyte PLA_2R epitope there begins a positive reinforcement with ever-increasing affinity. The exact nature of how patients eventually develop a pathogenic IgG antibody remains elusive. However, there is now tentative emerging evidence showing that in a control group of healthy volunteers and a patient group with active disease there is a PLA_2R antigen positive B cell population in both. This is coupled with an on-going unpublished study showing a level of circulating anti-PLA_2R IgM antibodies in these normal healthy patients. This requires further work, but it is the first evidence for an antibody class switch in autoimmune MN.

There is also data showing that as the anti-PLA_2R antibody rises in the weeks following treatment, there is a reduction in the natural T Regs. Following this, as the level of T Regs starts to rise there is a corresponding fall in the antibody level. Taken in tandem with unpublished work that is on-going showing a measurable level of circulating soluble PLA_2R in healthy controls, this would appear to show that a similar process to autoimmune thyroiditis is taking place in autoimmune MN.

There do remain a number of important questions in relation to the disease pathogenesis though; how does the anti-PLA_2R attaching to the epitope causes the damage we see? Despite strong circumstantial evidence suggesting its pathogenicity, direct evidence is currently lacking. Can the antibody titre supplant the need for a renal biopsy? How many patients who have the genetic predisposition eventually go on to develop the disease and is there a way to predict which patient does? And are there more autoantibodies associated with the development of autoimmune membranous nephropathy.

Current understanding of the role anti-PLA_2R plays in the pathogenesis has now led many to envisage a greater role for its use in clinical practice. Not only is it increasingly being used for disease monitoring and for prognosticating treatment response but it is also becoming a necessary tool for diagnosis. This has the distinct prospect of drastically altering the current diagnostic pathway and ultimately a patients quality of life. A number of groups are now actively investigating the feasibility of serum anti-PLA_2R negating the need for a renal biopsy, not only reducing time to diagnosis but also avoiding the need for an invasive procedure.

The hope is that by understanding the pathway of disease in this and other autoimmune conditions, new safer and more efficacious treatment options will be available for patients in the future. This is particularly pertinent given the increasing incidence of autoimmune diseases worldwide and the increased burden on patients and healthcare systems.

Author details

Patrick Hamilton[1,2,3*], Durga Kanigicherla[1,2] and Paul Brenchley[1,2,3]

1 Manchester Institute of Nephrology and Transplantation, Manchester Royal Infirmary, Manchester, United Kingdom

2 Manchester Academic Health Science Centre (MAHSC), The University of Manchester, Manchester, United Kingdom

3 Lydia Becker Institute of Immunology & Inflammation, The University of Manchester, Manchester, United Kingdom

*Address all correspondence to: patrick.hamilton@mft.nhs.uk

References

[1] TADC Committee. Progress in autoimmune diseases research. National Institutes of Health. 2005;**1**(1):1-146

[2] Cooper GS, Bynum MLK, Somers EC. Recent insights in the epidemiology of autoimmune diseases: Improved prevalence estimates and understanding of clustering of diseases. Journal of Autoimmunity. 2009;**33**(3-4):197-207

[3] McGrogan A, Franssen CFM, de Vries CS. The incidence of primary glomerulonephritis worldwide: A systematic review of the literature. Nephrology, Dialysis, Transplantation. 2011;**26**(2):414-430

[4] Barbour SJ, Greenwald A, Djurdjev O, Levin A, Hladunewich MA, Nachman PH, et al. Disease-specific risk of venous thromboembolic events is increased in idiopathic glomerulonephritis. Kidney International. 2011;**81**(2):190-195

[5] Llach F. Hypercoagulability, renal vein thrombosis, and other thrombotic complications of nephrotic syndrome. Kidney International. 1985;**28**(3):429-439

[6] Singhal R, Brimble KS. Thromboembolic complications in the nephrotic syndrome: Pathophysiology and clinical management. Thrombosis Research. 2006;**118**(3):397-407

[7] Eknoyan G, Eckardt KU, Kasiske BL. KDIGO clinical practice guideline for glomerulonephritis. Kidney International. 2012;**2**:143

[8] Schieppati A, Mosconi L, Perna A. Prognosis of untreated patients with idiopathic membranous nephropathy. The New England Journal of Medicine. 8 Jul 1993;**329**(2):85-89

[9] Wyld M, Morton RL, Hayen A, Howard K, Webster AC. A systematic review and meta-analysis of utility-based quality of life in chronic kidney disease treatments. PLoS Medicine. 2012;**9**(9):e1001307-e1001310

[10] Overbeck I, Bartels M, Decker O, Harms J. Changes in quality of life after renal transplantation. Transplantation Proceedings. Apr 2005;**37**(3):1618-1621. PubMed PMID: 15866689

[11] Schnuelle P, Lorenz D, Trede M, van der Woude FJ. Impact of renal cadaveric transplantation on survival in end-stage renal failure: Evidence for reduced mortality risk compared with hemodialysis during long-term follow-up. Journal of the American Society of Nephrology. 1998;**9**(11):2135-2141

[12] Moroni G, Gallelli B, Quaglini S, Leoni A, Banfi G, Passerini P, et al. Long-term outcome of renal transplantation in patients with idiopathic membranous glomerulonephritis (MN). Nephrology, Dialysis, Transplantation. 2010;**25**(10):3408-3415

[13] Doi T, Mayumi M, Kanatsu K, Suehiro F, Hamashima Y. Distribution of IgG subclasses in membranous nephropathy. Clinical and Experimental Immunology. 1984;**58**(1):57

[14] Oliveira DB. Membranous nephropathy: An IgG4-mediated disease. Lancet. 1998;**351**(9103):670-671

[15] Beck LH Jr, Bonegio RGB, Lambeau G, Beck DM, Powell DW, Cummins TD, et al. M-type phospholipase A 2receptor as target antigen in idiopathic membranous nephropathy. The New England Journal of Medicine. 2009;**361**(1):11-21

[16] Huang CC, Lehman A, Albawardi A, Satoskar A, Brodsky S, Nadasdy G, et al. IgG subclass staining in renal biopsies with membranous

glomerulonephritis indicates subclass switch during disease progression. Modern Pathology. 2013;**26**(6):799-805

[17] Vidarsson G, Dekkers G, Rispens T. IgG subclasses and allotypes: from structure to effector functions. Frontiers in Immunology. 20 Oct 2014;**5**:520. DOI: 10.3389/fimmu.2014.00520

[18] Ponticelli C, Zucchelli P, Passerini P, Cesana B, Locatelli F, Pasquali S, et al. A 10-year follow-up of a randomized study with methylprednisolone and chlorambucil in membranous nephropathy. Kidney International. 1995;**48**(5):1600-1604

[19] Ponticelli C, Altieri P, Scolari F, Passerini P, Roccatello D, Cesana B, et al. A randomized study comparing methylprednisolone plus chlorambucil versus methylprednisolone plus cyclophosphamide in idiopathic membranous nephropathy. Journal of the American Society of Nephrology. 1998;**9**(3):444-450

[20] Jha V, Ganguli A, Saha TK, Kohli HS, Sud K, Gupta KL, et al. A randomized, controlled trial of steroids and cyclophosphamide in adults with nephrotic syndrome caused by idiopathic membranous nephropathy. Journal of the American Society of Nephrology. 2007;**18**(6):1899-1904

[21] Cravedi P, Ruggenenti P, Remuzzi G. Circulating anti-PLA2R autoantibodies to monitor immunological activity in membranous nephropathy. Journal of the American Society of Nephrology. 2011;**22**(8):1400-1402

[22] Remuzzi G, Chiurchiu C, Abbate M, Brusegan V, Bontempelli M, Ruggenenti P. Rituximab for idiopathic membranous nephropathy. Lancet. 2002;**360**(9337):923-924

[23] Ruggenenti P, Cravedi P, Chianca A, Perna A, Ruggiero B, Gaspari F, et al. Rituximab in idiopathic membranous nephropathy. Journal of the American Society of Nephrology. 2012;**23**(8):1416-1425

[24] Dahan K, Debiec H, Plaisier E, Cachanado M, Rousseau A, Wakselman L, et al. Rituximab for severe membranous nephropathy: A 6-month trial with extended follow-up. Journal of the American Society of Nephrology. Jan 2017;**28**(1):348-358

[25] Hamilton P, Kanigicherla D, Venning M, Brenchley P, Meads D. Rituximab versus the modified Ponticelli regimen in the treatment of primary membranous nephropathy: A health economic model. Nephrology, Dialysis, Transplantation. 1 Dec 2018;**33**(12):2145-2155

[26] Belak M, Borberg H, Jimenez C, Oette K. Technical and clinical experience with protein A immunoadsorption columns. Transfusion Science. 1994;**15**(4):419-422

[27] Schwenger V, Morath C. Immunoadsorption in nephrology and kidney transplantation. Nephrology, Dialysis, Transplantation. 2010;**25**(8):2407-2413

[28] Müller J, Wallukat G, Dandel M, Bieda H, Brandes K, Spiegelsberger S, et al. Immunoglobulin adsorption in patients with idiopathic dilated cardiomyopathy. Circulation. 2000;**101**(4):385-391

[29] Dandel M, Wallukat G, Englert A, Hetzer R. Immunoadsorption therapy for dilated cardiomyopathy and pulmonary arterial hypertension. Atherosclerosis. Supplements. 2013;**14**(1):203-211

[30] Short CD, Feehally J, Gokal R, Mallick NP. Familial membranous nephropathy. British Medical Journal (Clinical Research Ed.). 1984;**289**(6457):1500

[31] Esnault VL, Besnier D, Testa A, Coville P, Simon P, Subra JF, et al. Effect of protein A immunoadsorption in nephrotic syndrome of various etiologies. Journal of the American Society of Nephrology. 1999;**10**(9):2014-2017

[32] Haas M, Godfrin Y, Oberbauer R, Yilmaz N, Borchhardt K, Regele H, et al. Plasma immunadsorption treatment in patients with primary focal and segmental glomerulosclerosis. Nephrology, Dialysis, Transplantation. 1998;**13**(8):2013-2016

[33] Stummvoll GH. Immunoadsorption (IAS) for systemic lupus erythematosus. Lupus. 2011;**20**(2):115-119

[34] Gaubitz M, Seidel M, Kummer S, Schotte H, Perniok A, Domschke W, et al. Prospective randomized trial of two different immunoadsorbers in severe systemic lupus erythematosus. Journal of Autoimmunity. 1998;**11**(5):495-501

[35] Koch M, Kohnle M, Trapp RA. Case report of successful long-term relapse control by protein-A immunoadsorption in an immunosuppressive-treated patient with end-stage renal disease due to Wegener's granulomatosis. Therapeutic Apheresis and Dialysis. 2009;**13**(2):150-156

[36] Matic G, Michelsen A, Hofmann D, Winkler R, Tiess M, Schneidewind JM, et al. Three cases of C-ANCA-positive vasculitis treated with immunoadsorption: Possible benefit in early treatment. Therapeutic Apheresis and Dialysis. 2001;**5**(1):68-72

[37] Biesenbach P, Kain R, Derfler K, Perkmann T, Soleiman A, Benharkou A, et al. Long-term outcome of anti-glomerular basement membrane antibody disease treated with immunoadsorption. PLoS One. 2014;**9**(7):e103568

[38] Higgins RM, Bevan DJ, Carey BS, Lea CK, Fallon M, Bühler R, et al. Prevention of hyperacute rejection by removal of antibodies to HLA immediately before renal transplantation. Lancet. 1996;**348**(9036):1208-1211

[39] Haas M, Böhmig GA, Mohr ZL, Exner M, Regele H, Derfler K, et al. Peri-operative immunoadsorption in sensitized renal transplant recipients. Nephrology, Dialysis, Transplantation. 2002;**17**(8):1503-1508

[40] Böhmig GA, Regele H, Exner M, Derhartunian V, Kletzmayr J, Säemann MD, et al. C4d-positive acute humoral renal allograft rejection: Effective treatment by immunoadsorption. Journal of the American Society of Nephrology. 2001;**12**(11):2482-2489

[41] Farquhar MG, Saito A, Kerjaschki D, Orlando RA. The Heymann nephritis antigenic complex: Megalin (gp330) and RAP. Journal of the American Society of Nephrology. 1995;**6**(1):35-47

[42] Kerjaschki D, Farquhar MG. The pathogenic antigen of Heymann nephritis is a membrane glycoprotein of the renal proximal tubule brush border. Proceedings of the National Academy of Sciences of the United States of America. 1982;**79**(18):5557-5561

[43] Jefferson JA, Pippin JW, Shankland SJ. Experimental models of membranous nephropathy. Drug Discovery Today: Disease Models. 2010;**7**(1-2):27-33

[44] Tomas NM, Beck LH Jr, Meyer-Schwesinger C, Seitz-Polski B, Ma H, Zahner G, et al. Thrombospondin type-1 domain-containing 7A in idiopathic membranous nephropathy. The New England Journal of Medicine. 2014;**371**(24):2277-2287

[45] Beck LH Jr. The dominant humoral epitope in phospholipase A2 receptor-1: Presentation matters when serving up a slice of π. Journal of

the American Society of Nephrology. 2015;**26**(2):237-239

[46] East L. The mannose receptor family. Biochimica et Biophysica Acta (BBA). 2002;**1572**(2-3):364-386

[47] Llorca O. Extended and bent conformations of the mannose receptor family. Cellular and Molecular Life Sciences. 2008;**65**(9):1302-1310

[48] Fresquet M, Jowitt TA, Gummadova J, Collins R, O'Cualain R, McKenzie EA, et al. Identification of a major epitope recognized by PLA2R autoantibodies in primary membranous nephropathy. Journal of the American Society of Nephrology. Feb 2015;**26**(2):302-313

[49] Granata F, Petraroli A, Boilard E, Bezzine S, Bollinger J, Del Vecchio L, et al. Activation of cytokine production by secreted phospholipase A2 in human lung macrophages expressing the M-type receptor. Journal of Immunology. 2005;**174**(1):464-474

[50] Silliman CC, Moore EE, Zallen G, Gonzalez R, Johnson JL, Elzi DJ, et al. Presence of the M-type sPLA2 receptor on neutrophils and its role in elastase release and adhesion. American Journal of Physiology-Cell Physiology. 2002;**283**(4):C1102-C1113

[51] Herrmann SMS, Sethi S, Fervenza FC. Membranous nephropathy. Current Opinion in Nephrology and Hypertension. 2012;**21**(2):203-210

[52] Hoxha E, Kneißler U, Stege G, Zahner G, Thiele I, Panzer U, et al. Enhanced expression of the M-type phospholipase A2 receptor in glomeruli correlates with serum receptor antibodies in primary membranous nephropathy. Kidney International. 2012;**82**(7):797-804

[53] Kerjaschki D, Miettinen A, Farquhar MG. Initial events in the formation of immune deposits in passive Heymann nephritis. gp330-anti-gp330 immune complexes form in epithelial coated pits and rapidly become attached to the glomerular basement membrane. The Journal of Experimental Medicine. 1987;**166**(1):109-128

[54] Debiec H, Ronco P. PLA2R autoantibodies and PLA2R glomerular deposits in membranous nephropathy. The New England Journal of Medicine. 2011;**364**(7):689-690

[55] Kanigicherla D, Gummadova J, McKenzie EA, Roberts SA, Harris S, Nikam M, et al. Anti-PLA2R antibodies measured by ELISA predict long-term outcome in a prevalent population of patients with idiopathic membranous nephropathy. Kidney International. 2013;**83**(5):940-948

[56] Hofstra JM, Laurence H, Beck J, Beck DM, Wetzels JF, Salant DJ. Anti-phospholipase A2 receptor antibodies correlate with clinical status in idiopathic membranous nephropathy. Clinical Journal of the American Society of Nephrology. 2011;**6**(6):1286-1291

[57] Bech AP, Hofstra JM, Brenchley PE, Wetzels JFM. Association of anti-PLA2R antibodies with outcomes after immunosuppressive therapy in idiopathic membranous nephropathy. Clinical Journal of the American Society of Nephrology. 2014;**9**(8):1386-1392

[58] Beck LH, Fervenza FC, Beck DM, Bonegio RGB, Malik FA, Erickson SB, et al. Rituximab-induced depletion of anti-PLA2R autoantibodies predicts response in membranous nephropathy. Journal of the American Society of Nephrology. 2011;**22**(8):1543-1550

[59] Ruggenenti P, Debiec H, Ruggiero B, Chianca A, Pellé T, Gaspari F, et al. Anti-phospholipase A2 receptor antibody titer predicts post-rituximab outcome of membranous nephropathy. Journal of the American Society of Nephrology. 2015;**26**(10):2545-2558

[60] Hoxha E, Thiele I, Zahner G, Panzer U, Harendza S, Stahl RAK. Phospholipase

A2 receptor autoantibodies and clinical outcome in patients with primary membranous nephropathy. Journal of the American Society of Nephrology. 2014;**25**(6):1357-1366

[61] Kao L, Lam V, Waldman M, Glassock RJ, Zhu Q. Identification of the immunodominant epitope region in phospholipase A2 receptor-mediating autoantibody binding in idiopathic membranous nephropathy. Journal of the American Society of Nephrology. 2015;**26**(2):291-301

[62] Seitz-Polski B, Dolla G, Payré C, Girard CA, Polidori J, Zorzi K, et al. Epitope spreading of autoantibody response to PLA2R associates with poor prognosis in membranous nephropathy. Journal of the American Society of Nephrology. 2016;**27**(5):1517-1533

[63] Müller GA, Müller C, Liebau G, Kömpf J, Ising H, Wernet P. strong association of idiopathic membranous nephropathy (IMN) with HLA-DR 3 and MT-2 without involvement of HLA-B 18 and no Association to BfF1. Tissue Antigens. 1981;**17**(3):332-337

[64] Klouda PT, Manos J, Acheson EJ, Dyer PA, Goldby FS, Harris R, et al. Strong association between idiopathic membranous nephropathy and HLA-DRW3. Lancet. 1979;**2**(8146):770-771

[65] Kim S, Chin HJ, Na KY, Kim S, Oh J, Chung W, et al. Single nucleotide polymorphisms in the phospholipase A2 receptor gene are associated with genetic susceptibility to idiopathic membranous nephropathy. Nephron. Clinical Practice. 2011;**117**(3):c253-c258

[66] Liu Y-H, Chen C-H, Chen S-Y, Lin Y-J, Liao W-L, Tsai C-H, et al. Association of phospholipase A2 receptor 1 polymorphisms with idiopathic membranous nephropathy in Chinese patients in Taiwan. Journal of Biomedical Science. 2010;**17**(1):81

[67] Stanescu HC, Arcos-Burgos M, Medlar A, Bockenhauer D, Köttgen A, Dragomirescu L, et al. Risk HLA-DQA1 and PLA(2)R1 alleles in idiopathic membranous nephropathy. The New England Journal of Medicine. 2011;**364**(7):616-626

[68] Sekula P, Li Y, Stanescu HC, Wuttke M, Ekici AB, Bockenhauer D, et al. Genetic risk variants for membranous nephropathy: Extension of and association with other chronic kidney disease aetiologies. Nephrology, Dialysis, Transplantation. 2017;**32**(2):325-332

[69] Altschul SF, Madden TL, Schäffer AA, Zhang J, Zhang Z, Miller W, et al. Gapped BLAST and PSI-BLAST: A new generation of protein database search programs. Nucleic Acids Research. Oxford University Press. 1997;**25**(17):3389-3402

[70] Kong Y, Brown N, Morris G, Flynn J. The essential role of circulating thyroglobulin in maintaining dominance of natural regulatory T cell function to prevent autoimmune thyroiditis. Hormone and Metabolic Research. 2015;**47**(10):711-720

[71] Rosenzwajg M, Languille E, Debiec H, Hygino J, Dahan K, Simon T, et al. B- and T-cell subpopulations in patients with severe idiopathic membranous nephropathy may predict an early response to rituximab. Kidney International. Jul 2017;**92**(1):227-237. DOI: 10.1016/j.kint.2017.01.012

[72] Hamilton P, Kanigicherla D, Hanumapura P, Walz L, Kramer D, Fischer M, et al. Peptide GAM immunoadsorption therapy in primary membranous nephropathy (PRISM): Phase II trial investigating the safety and feasibility of peptide GAM immunoadsorption in anti-PLA 2R positive primary membranous nephropathy. Journal of Clinical Apheresis. 2017;**17**(9):1594-1598

Chapter 6

Treatment of Idiopathic Membranous Nephropathy (IMN)

María Carmen Prados Soler, María Dolores Del Pino y Pino, Álvaro Pérez Fernández, Llenalia Gordillo García, María José López Ruiz and César Luis Ramírez-Tortosa

Abstract

We present a 59-year-old patient with type 2 diabetes mellitus and massive nephrotic syndrome (anasarca) and biochemical syndrome. The renal biopsy showed a membranous nephropathy (MN). In the blood analysis the patient presented antibodies against M-type phospholipase A2 receptor (anti-PLA2R) positive at a very high titer. Given the existence of idiopathic membranous nephropathy (IMN), treatment was started with a modified Ponticelli regimen, with no response, requiring periodic ultrafiltration sessions. Rituximab induces nephrotic syndrome (NS) remission in two-thirds of patients with IMN, even after other treatments have failed. We proposed treatment with rituximab based on published evidence. In IMN, the presence of M-type anti-receptor antibodies of A2 phospholipase is considered highly specific to idiopathic forms, but the presence of such antibodies has not been shown to be associated with a particular clinical profile. Assessing circulating anti-PLA2R autoantibodies and proteinuria may help in monitoring disease activity and guiding personalized rituximab therapy in nephrotic patients with IMN.

Keywords: idiopathic membranous nephropathy, nephrotic syndrome, antibodies against M-type phospholipase A2 receptor (anti-PLA2R), rituximab

1. Introduction

MN is a disease characterized by the deposition of immune complexes at subepithelial level. Its most frequent clinical presentation is NS, and it is today the first cause of NS in the Caucasian adult [1].

In recent years, it has been discovered that IMN has an immunological basis. The data in favour of this alteration of the immune system are the findings found in the electron microscopy of renal biopsies, the granular deposits of immunoglobulin G (mainly IgG4) and C3 along the glomerular basement membrane, and the deposit of electrodense immunocomplexes in the subepithelium that entails an activation of the complement products. MN may also be secondary to infections, tumors, autoimmune diseases, and use of different drugs [1]. PLA2R has been found to be the target antigen of autoantibodies in IMN patients, and is known as anti-PLA2R. PLA2R is a type I transmembrane glycoprotein related to the animal family of type C lectin. More recently, anti-PLA2Rs have been found to be immunoglobulins of the IgG4 type [2]. Currently, these antibodies are present in 60–80%

IntechOpen

of IMN patients prior to immunosuppressive therapy. However, in secondary MN forms these antibodies are much less prevalent. No anti-PLA2R has been observed in other pathological conditions or in healthy individuals. In recent years, articles have been published in which several researchers have addressed the appearance of anti-PLA2R antibodies in patients with secondary MN, so more data are needed to conclude with certainty that when these antibodies are found, there is no need to investigate an underlying cause to guide a secondary MN [2, 3].

Recently, various studies have described that about 70% of MNI cases are associated with the presence of anti-PLA2R. Antibody titer at diagnosis is related to the likelihood of spontaneous remission (SR) and response to treatment. However, it has not been demonstrated that in patients with MNI, the presence of anti-PLA2R antibodies is associated with a certain clinical profile of disease presentation or implies differences in clinical course, response to treatment or long-term prognosis. On the other hand, although most studies agree that the presence of anti-PLA2R antibodies is highly specific to IMN, there are cases described in which the presence of these antibodies coincides with other possible etiologies and about 30% of patients with IMN are anti-PLA2R negative. In this last group of patients, antibodies have been described against other podocyte antigens whose clinical correlation is still being investigated and, therefore, there is greater uncertainty about the possible identification of secondary etiologies over time. However, since most studies have been cross-sectional, little information is available about the diagnosis of possible etiologies responsible for MN over time in both positive and negative anti-PLA2R patients [4].

In IMN the disease appears to develop by the binding of an autoantibody directed against an antigen. A podocyte that is located on the subepithelial slope of the podocyte. For this motive there are currently various immunosuppressive treatments available [2].

A very high percentage of patients (more than 40% in many series) develop spontaneous remission of the disease without any type of treatment, while another considerable percentage (around 30–40%) develops progressive renal failure accompanied by nephrotic proteinuria [2].

Ponticelli in 1989 showed that combined treatment with cytotoxics produced partial or complete remission of proteinuria in a significant proportion of patients with membranous nephropathy [5]. However, the literature is controversial regarding the effectiveness of the scheme described by Ponticelli et al. [6].

The most important predictors of risk for a progressive decline in renal function are persistent severe proteinuria for at least 3 months, a reduced creatinine clearance at presentation, and a decline in creatinine clearance over the assessed proteinuria period [7].

Resistant patients are defined as those with moderate or high risk disease who fail an adequate trial of treatment with both cyclophosphamide-based and calcineurin inhibitor-based regimens [8].

A trial of rituximab can be considered after a careful evaluation of the potential risks and benefits of further immunosuppression. Weak evidence suggests that a clinically relevant response to rituximab may be less likely in patients with a creatinine clearance below 75 mL/min per 1.73 m^2 [9].

In this case, we present a 59-year-old patient with type 2 diabetes mellitus and massive nephrotic syndrome (anasarca) and biochemical syndrome. The renal biopsy showed a membranous nephropathy (MN). Anti-PLA2 positive antibodies at a very high titer (366 RU/mL). Given the existence of IMN, treatment was started with a modified Ponticelli regimen, with no response, requiring periodic ultrafiltration sessions. We proposed treatment with rituximab based on published evidence.

2. Clinical case

A 59-year-old male with a history of long-standing type 2 DM with retinopathy and diabetic neuropathy, OSAS and intrinsic asthma. Blood pressure and normal renal function. One month prior to your entry into our Service (October 2018) refers pretibial edemas—malleolar and scrotal edema of morning onset, with worsening throughout the day and dyspnea of moderate efforts. Initially consult with your Primary Care doctor, being treated with furosemide. In the absence of a response, he is referred to the hospital.

Upon admission, the patient is afebrile, dyspnoeic, conscious and oriented and presents a slight cutaneous-mucosal pallor. Blood pressure: 100/70 mmHg. Heart rate: 72 bpm. Normal head, neck without jugular vein. Rhythmic cardiac auscultation, without murmurs. Respiratory auscultation with bilateral diffuse crackles. Abdomen, without pathological findings and lower extremities with edemas ++++/++++ to English that leave fovea. Scrotal edema. No signs of deep vein thrombosis. Peripheral pulses preserved. Analytical on admission: leukocytes 7.30 × 10. e3/μL with normal formula, hemoglobin 11 g/dl, hematocrit 32.5%, platelets 164 × 10.3/μL ESR 19 mm/h, sodium 138 mM/L, potassium 3.9 mM/L, urea 110 mg/dl, creatinine 2.08 mg/dl, total cholesterol 282 mg/dl, cholesterol-HDL 88 mg/ml cholesterol-LDL 158 mg/ml, triglycerides 171 mg/dl, albumin 2.4 g/dl, total protein 4.9 g/dl. GOT, GPT, LDH, GGT, alkaline phosphatase, glucose, calcium, phosphorus and bilirubin within normal limits. Protein level in blood: albumin 44.2%, alpha-1 9.4%, alpha-2 17.4%, beta 18.2%, gamma 10.7%. In urine: proteinuria 14 g/24 h. Coagulation: normal, fibrinogen 676. Tumor markers: carcinoembryonic antigen, alpha-fetoprotein, PSA ng/ml and Ca 19.9: normal. ANA, ANCA, rheumatoid factor and negative glomerular baseline anti-membrane antibodies. NT-ProBNP: 200 pg/ml. Ac anti-PLA2: positive (366 RU/mL).

Kidney ultrasound showed normal-sized kidneys, with good cortico-medullary differentiation, without dilation of the urinary tract. A percutaneous renal biopsy was performed observing a renal parenchyma corresponding to the cortical zone that included 28 glomeruli. Diffuse and global thickening of the glomerular basement membranes by subepithelial deposit ("comb peaks") with mesangial focal extension not associated with mesangial cell proliferation but with floccular-capsular adhesions, no endocapillary proliferation or glomerulitis, absence of

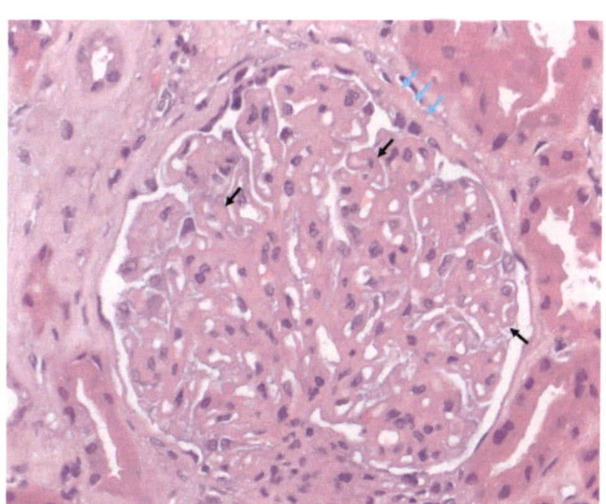

Figure 1.
Staining with Hematoxylin and Eosin. 40X, Global Thickening of the capillary membranes (black arrows) of the glomerulus not accompanied by mesangial or endocapillary proliferation. Discreet thickening of Bowman's capsule (blue arrow).

karyorrhexis, irregular thickening of Bowman's capsule, immunocomplex subepithelial deposits (IgG), Glomerular sclerosis (10%); tubular atrophy and interstitial fibrosis (moderate), arteriosclerosis (moderate), hyaline arteriolosclerosis, and vascular changes associated with hypertension (**Figures 1–6**). Depletive treatment

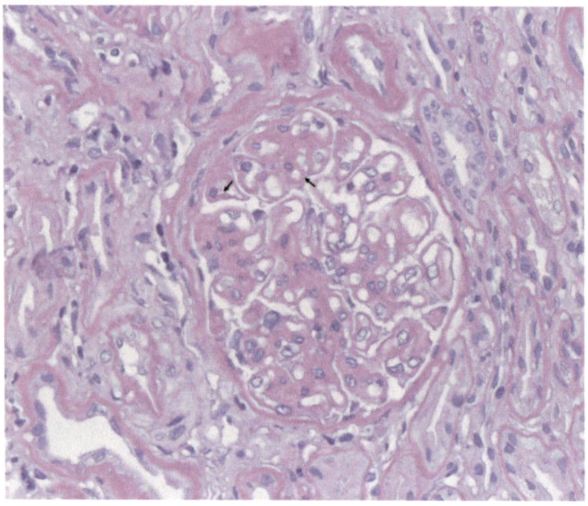

Figure 2.
PAS 40X. The technique of PAS also shows the thickening of glomerular capillary membranes (black arrows).

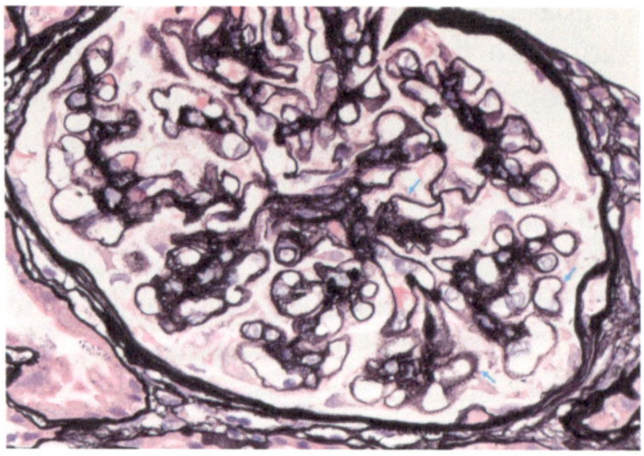

Figure 3.
Jones' Silver. 40X. subepithelial Depsoits in the basal membranes of the glomerular capillaries showing an image in "Spikes de peine" (blue Arrow). This technique stains the basal membrane black. Immuncomplements deposits are not stained.

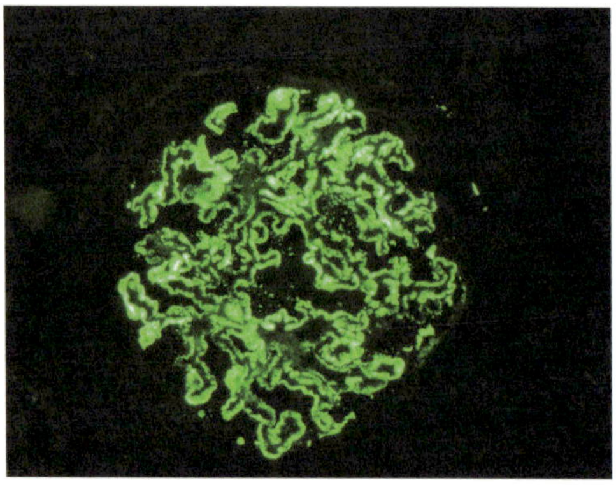

Figure 4.
IF. IgG. Subepithelial granular Deposits in capillary basal membrane with global and diffuse pattern and staining intensity 3 +/3.

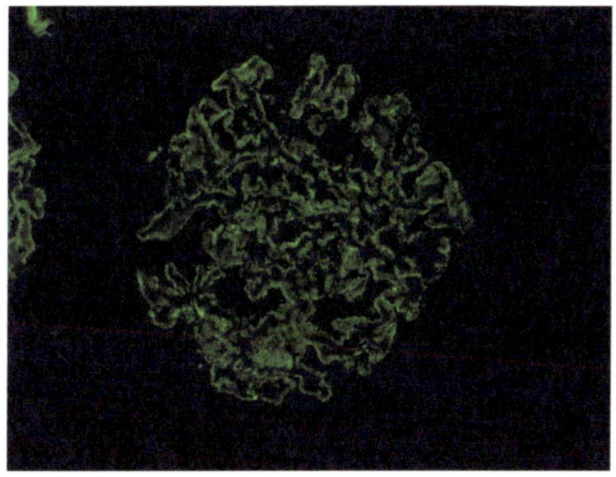

Figure 5.
IF. Lambda Light Chains. Subepithelial granular Deposits in capillary basal membrane with global and diffuse pattern and staining intensity 1-2 +/3.

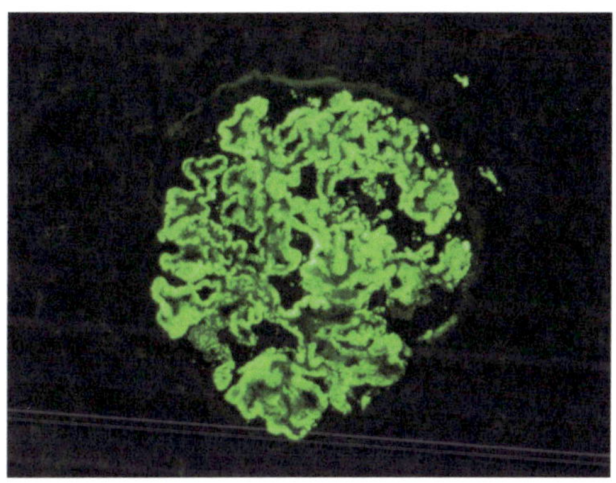

Figure 6.
IF. Kappa Light Chains. Subepithelial granular Deposits in capillary basal membrane with global and diffuse pattern and staining intensity 3 +/3.

was started with IV furosemide at high doses and IV albumin, with poor response, requiring periodic ultrafiltration sessions. Treatment was started with a modified Ponticelli regimen: prednisone at a dose of 0.5 mg/kg/day and cyclophosphamide 125 mg/day initially and then 100 mg/day, adjusted for renal function. An inhibitor of the angiotensin conversion enzyme was associated. Two months later, proteinuria has not changed. Kidney function remains normal. After 2 months of treatment, we have not shown changes in proteinuria. Continue to specify ultrafiltration sessions. We have decided to administer Rituximab. We will continue to monitor renal function, proteinuria and anti-PLA2 Ac.

3. Discussion

MN is the first cause of NS in the adult [1]. From A clinical perspective, it is classified in idiopathic (IMN) or secondary depending on whether or not it is possible to identify a responsible etiology. In the absence of clinical or biochemical data indicating a specific etiology, distinguishing between the two forms can be difficult only through the data provided by the renal biopsy [2].

MN in adults is most often idiopathic (approximately 75% of cases) but can be caused by a variety of drugs, infections, and underlying diseases. These include gold, penicillamine, systemic lupus erythematosus, malignancy, and hepatitis B and C virus infection [2].

It is often not possible to distinguish idiopathic from secondary MN on clinical grounds alone, even though serologic studies (e.g., antinuclear antibodies, hepatitis B serology) and a history of drug exposure or cancer may be revealing of a potential cause. However, there are certain findings on electron microscopy and immunofluorescence that suggest secondary disease. In patients with secondary MN, cessation of the offending drug or effective treatment of the underlying disease is usually associated with improvement in the nephrotic syndrome [10].

In view of the potential toxicity of the drugs used to treat IMN, with or without the nephrotic syndrome, the decision to initiate therapy is based, in part, upon an understanding of the natural history of untreated patients, with and without features of the nephrotic syndrome at presentation [11]:

- Spontaneous complete remission of proteinuria occurs in 5–30% at 5 years.
- Spontaneous partial remission (≤2 g of proteinuria per day) occurs in 25–40% at 5 years.
- The occurrence of end-stage renal disease in untreated patients is approximately 14% at 5 years, 35% at 10 years, and 41% at 15 years.

Risk factors for progressive idiopathic MN—in view of the often benign clinical course, immunosuppressive agents should be considered only in those with idiopathic MN who are most at risk for progressive disease or who have severe symptomatic nephrotic syndrome. Both histologic and clinical findings may be important in risk assessment.

- Clinical findings associated with a higher risk of developing end-stage renal disease include older age at onset (particularly greater than 50 years), male sex, nephrotic-range proteinuria (particularly if protein excretion exceeds 8–10 g/day), and an increased serum creatinine at presentation [12].

In contrast to these adverse risk factors, women, children, and young adults, non-nephrotic-range proteinuria, a progressive decline in protein excretion, and presentation with normal renal function have been associated with a relatively benign course [7]. In addition, patients of Asian ancestry seem to have a better long-term prognosis than other ancestries.

- Histologic findings are frequently regarded as important predictors of outcome, as the risk of progression is increased in patients with glomerular scarring (segmental sclerosis) and correlates more closely with the severity of the tubulointerstitial disease than with the degree of glomerular injury [12, 13]. This observation is typical of most glomerular diseases.

Importance of attaining remission—attainment of a complete remission (whether spontaneous or not) is associated with good long-term outcomes. In contrast, little is known about the prognosis in patients with a partial remission [14].

A complete remission was defined as protein excretion below 0.3 g/day, while a partial remission was defined as protein excretion below 3.5 g/day plus a 50% or greater reduction in protein excretion from the peak value. Renal failure was defined as a creatinine clearance ≤15 mL/min, initiation of dialysis, or renal transplantation.

The following findings were associated with a better renal survival on multivariate analysis that took into account clinical and laboratory data:

- higher initial creatinine clearance and lower proteinuria at presentation,
- lower mean arterial blood pressure over the observation period,
- attainment of complete or partial remission in proteinuria.

Based upon this model, is defined as low-, moderate-, and high-risk patient subsets with varying degrees of risk for progression to more advanced kidney insufficiency (defined as a creatinine clearance ≤60 mL/min per 1.73 m^2) over 5 years:

- Low risk—proteinuria remains less than 4 g/day and creatinine clearance remains normal for a 6-month follow-up period. Such patients have a less than 8% risk of developing chronic renal insufficiency over 5 years.
- Moderate risk—proteinuria is between 4 and 8 g/day and persists for more than 6 months. Creatinine clearance is normal or near normal and remains stable over 6 months of observation. Chronic renal insufficiency develops over 5 years in approximately 50% of these patients.
- High risk—proteinuria is greater than 8 g/day and persists for 3 months and/or renal function that is either below normal (and considered due to MN) or decreases during the observation period. Approximately 75% of such patients are at risk of progression to chronic renal insufficiency over 5 years.

4. Nonimmunosuppressive therapies

Given the high rate of gradual spontaneous improvement in patients with IMN, only selected patients with more severe or progressive disease should receive immunosuppressive therapy [1].

In contrast, almost all patients are candidates for more general therapies for nephrotic syndrome, such as angiotensin inhibition, lipid lowering, and, in selected patients, anticoagulation. Other aspects of therapy include diuretics to control edema and maintenance of adequate nutrition.

Proteinuria goal—the optimal proteinuria goal in patients with chronic kidney disease is less than 1000 mg/day. However, this goal is often not attainable in patients with IMN.

Goal blood pressure—the goal blood pressure in patients with MN is the same as it is in other patients with proteinuric chronic kidney disease (125/75 mmHg). Attainment of this goal can slow the progression of proteinuric chronic kidney disease and can provide cardiovascular protection since chronic kidney disease is associated with a marked increase in cardiovascular risk. The data supporting these recommendations are presented separately.

Attainment of the blood pressure goal in patients with MN usually requires more than angiotensin inhibition alone. Correction of volume overload is of particular importance and usually requires loop diuretics. Diuretics should be pushed until the blood pressure goal is reached or the patient has attained "dry weight" which, in the presence of persistent hypertension, is defined as the weight at which further fluid removal leads to symptoms (fatigue, orthostatic hypotension) or to decreased tissue perfusion as evidenced by an otherwise unexplained elevation in the blood urea nitrogen and/or serum creatinine concentration.

A low-salt diet is an important component of antihypertensive therapy (especially when using angiotensin inhibitors) and edema control in patients with MN. In addition, a high-salt diet can increase proteinuria, and in some individuals, a high-salt diet rather than increased immunologic activity should be considered as an underlying cause of worsening proteinuria.

Lipid lowering—hyperlipidemia, with often dramatic elevations in the serum cholesterol concentration, is commonly present in patients with nephrotic syndrome. The mainstay of therapy for such hypercholesterolemia is statins.

5. Immunosuppressive therapies

Indications for and choice of therapy—since many patients with mild to moderate disease undergo spontaneous remission and immunosuppressive agents have appreciable toxicity, the decision to treat must be based upon the probability that the patient will have progressive disease (defined as an otherwise unexplained elevation in serum creatinine or persistent high-grade or increasing proteinuria in patients at moderate to high risk for progression) [15].

The treatment regimen must be based upon the risk of progressive disease. First-line immunosuppressive therapy consists of cytotoxic drugs (usually cyclophosphamide) plus glucocorticoids or a calcineurin inhibitor with low-dose or no glucocorticoids (a regimen based upon cytotoxic drugs is preferred in some high-risk patients with declining glomerular filtration rate due to MN and an estimated glomerular filtration rate above 30 mL/min/1.73 m^2). Patients who do not respond to one regimen are usually treated with the other, and those with resistant disease may be treated with rituximab.

In our case, it is a patient with a high risk of progression.

High risk for progression—high-risk patients with idiopathic MN are defined as those with protein excretion exceeding 8 g/day that persists for more than 3 months and/or renal function that is either below normal (and considered due to MN) or decreases during the observation period, despite maximum nonimmunosuppressive therapy. These patients are also likely to have prominent nephrotic symptoms or signs, such as marked hypoalbuminemia and edema. Approximately 75% of such patients progress to worsened renal insufficiency over 5 years.

Rituximab has been used in patients with idiopathic membranous nephropathy who have failed previous treatment with other immunosuppressive regimens.

Rituximab may have benefit among patients with a moderate risk of progression who have not previously received immunosuppressive therapy [8, 16]. In one unblinded trial for 12 months, the rate of complete or partial remission was higher among patients treated with rituximab (65 versus 34%). These findings are consistent with observational studies that demonstrate a maximal reduction in proteinuria at 18–24 months after treatment with rituximab. Anti-PLA2R antibodies, which were present in 73% of patients at baseline, disappeared in a greater proportion of patients receiving rituximab (50 versus 12%). Serious adverse events were similar between the two groups.

Resistant disease—the optimal approach to moderate- or high-risk patients with stable renal function who fail treatment with both cyclophosphamide and calcineurin inhibitor-based regimens is not known. We prefer a trial of rituximab in such patients, although limited data are available suggesting efficacy.

Several observational (nonrandomized) studies in patients with idiopathic resistant MN have reported outcomes following the administration of rituximab:

Rituximab therapy is generally well tolerated, adverse effects are minor and primarily consisted of infusion reactions.

Anti-PLA2R-positive patients with lower titers had significantly greater remission rates compared with patients who had higher titers.

Rituximab may provide benefit to patients who failed prior immunosuppressive therapy, especially those with relatively preserved renal function. Four weekly doses of rituximab (375 mg/m^2) appear to have the same effect on proteinuria reduction as a regimen of 1 g every 2 weeks.

It is suggested the somewhat simpler and cheaper regimen of a dose of 1 g given intravenously and repeated in 2 weeks. Patients who continue to have significant proteinuria may have this dose repeated at 6 months.

PLA2R is a transmembrane receptor that is highly expressed in glomerular podocytes and has been identified as a major antigen in human idiopathic MN.

A decline in antiphospholipase A2 receptor (PLA2R) antibodies may predict the clinical response to rituximab treatment [17, 18].

The anti-PLA2R autoantibody-negative patients may be in the midst of a spontaneous or treatment-induced remission.

The monitoring serum anti-PLA2R antibodies may allow a more accurate assessment of the immunological response to rituximab (and possibly other therapies) than is provided by measurement of proteinuria alone [17, 18].

6. Conclusions

MN is among the most common causes of the nephrotic syndrome in nondiabetic adults, accounting for up to one-third of biopsy diagnoses.

A significant percentage (15–50% of cases) of patients with IMN develop progressive chronic kidney disease.

Rituximab induces NS remission in two-thirds of patients with IMN, even after other treatments have failed. The rate of complete or partial remission was higher among patients treated with Rituximab.

Therefore, assessing circulating anti-PLA2R autoantibodies and proteinuria may help in monitoring disease activity and guiding personalized rituximab therapy in nephrotic patients with IMN. The monitoring serum anti-PLA2R antibodies may allow a more accurate assessment of the immunological response to rituximab (and possibly other therapies) than is provided by measurement of proteinuria alone.

Author details

María Carmen Prados Soler[1*], María Dolores Del Pino y Pino[1], Álvaro Pérez Fernández[1], Llenalia Gordillo García[1], María José López Ruiz[1] and César Luis Ramírez-Tortosa[2]

1 Nephrology Service, Complejo Hospitalario Torrecárdenas, Almería, Spain

2 Pathological Anatomy Service, Hospital Virgen de las Nieves, Granada, Spain

*Address all correspondence to: lensasu@yahoo.es

References

[1] Fervenza FC, Sethi S, Specks U. Idiopathic membranous nephropathy: Diagnosis and treatment. Clinical Journal of the American Society of Nephrology. 2008;**3**:905

[2] Debiec H, Ronco P. PLA2R autoantibodies and PLA2R glomerular deposits in membranous nephropathy. The New England Journal of Medicine. 2011;**364**:689

[3] Qin W, Beck LH Jr, Zeng C, et al. Anti-phospholipase A2 receptor antibody in membranous nephropathy. Journal of the American Society of Nephrology. 2011;**22**:1137

[4] Hofstra JM, Beck LH Jr, Beck DM, et al. Anti-phospholipase A_2 receptor antibodies correlate with clinical status in idiopathic membranous nephropathy. Clinical Journal of the American Society of Nephrology. 2011;**6**:1286

[5] Ponticelli C, Zucchelli P, Passerini P, et al. A 10-year follow-up of a randomized study with methylprednisolone and chlorambucil in membranous nephropathy. Kidney International. 1995;**48**:1600

[6] Ponticelli C, Altieri P, Scolari F, et al. A randomized study comparing methylprednisolone plus chlorambucil versus methylprednisolone plus cyclophosphamide in idiopathic membranous nephropathy. Journal of the American Society of Nephrology. 1998;**9**:444

[7] Reichert LJ, Koene RA, Wetzels JF. Prognostic factors in idiopathic membranous nephropathy. American Journal of Kidney Diseases. 1998;**31**:1

[8] Dahan K, Debiec H, Plaisier E, et al. Rituximab for severe membranous nephropathy: A 6-month trial with extended follow-up. Journal of the American Society of Nephrology. 2017;**28**:348

[9] Ruggenenti P, Cravedi P, Chianca A, et al. Rituximab in idiopathic membranous nephropathy. Journal of the American Society of Nephrology. 2012;**23**:1416

[10] Troyanov S, Roasio L, Pandes M, et al. Renal pathology in idiopathic membranous nephropathy: A new perspective. Kidney International. 2006;**69**:1641

[11] Jha V, Ganguli A, Saha TK, et al. A randomized, controlled trial of steroids and cyclophosphamide in adults with nephrotic syndrome caused by idiopathic membranous nephropathy. Journal of the American Society of Nephrology. 2007;**18**:1899

[12] Shiiki H, Saito T, Nishitani Y, et al. Prognosis and risk factors for idiopathic membranous nephropathy with nephrotic syndrome in Japan. Kidney International. 2004;**65**:1400

[13] Wu Q, Jinde K, Nishina M, et al. Analysis of prognostic predictors in idiopathic membranous nephropathy. American Journal of Kidney Diseases. 2001;**37**:380

[14] Troyanov S, Wall CA, Miller JA, et al. Idiopathic membranous nephropathy: Definition and relevance of a partial remission. Kidney International. 2004;**66**:1199

[15] Philibert D, Cattran D. Remission of proteinuria in primary glomerulonephritis: We know the goal but do we know the price? Nature Clinical Practice. Nephrology. 2008;**4**:550

[16] Ruggenenti P, Debiec H, Ruggiero B, et al. Anti-phospholipase A2 receptor antibody titer predicts post-rituximab outcome of membranous nephropathy. Journal of the American Society of Nephrology. 2015;**26**:2545

[17] Cattran DC, Kim ED, Reich H, et al. Membranous nephropathy: Quantifying remission duration on outcome. Journal of the American Society of Nephrology. 2017;**28**:995

[18] Cravedi P, Ruggenenti P, Remuzzi G. Circulating anti-PLA2R autoantibodies to monitor immunological activity in membranous nephropathy. Journal of the American Society of Nephrology. 2011;**22**:1400

Section 4

Renal Rehabilitation

Chapter 7

Renal Rehabilitation: A Perspective From Human Body Movement

Jorge Enrique Moreno Collazos and Diana Carolina Zona Rubio

Abstract

The prevalence and incidence of advanced chronic kidney disease has grown progressively in most countries of the world. Hemodialysis is the most common treatment that replaces the renal function, and although it allows to replace the function of the kidney, the patients who undergo it can present numerous alterations that lead to a loss of functional physical capacity and a decrease in the quality of life related to health. It is unknown to what extent low physical activity, uremia and anemia determine the decrease in functional capacity of these patients. The functional tests most frequently used in the published literature are characterized by their ease of application and their low cost, since they do not require large measuring instruments to quantify basic qualities in subjects with impaired or dysfunction of the renal system from the aerobic capacity, muscle performance and flexibility as axes within the kinetic wellbeing which is committed in the stay of the renal hemodialysis units.

Keywords: rehabilitation, exercise, renal dialysis, physiotherapy

1. Introduction

Rehabilitation specialists currently perform in a variety of important intervention areas, positively diminishing the impact of various alterations, such as, renal dysfunction in hemodialysis care units [1]. Survival of patients with this disease at 5 years is 40% and the life expectancy of patients on dialysis is one fourth to one fifth of the general population [2]. Chronic kidney disease is becoming a serious health problem throughout the world and is one of the most known risk factors for cardiovascular disease, being this the main cause of morbidity and mortality in this patient population. On the other hand, physical inactivity has become a significant and independent risk factor for the accelerated deterioration of renal function, physical function, cardiovascular function and the quality of life of people in all stages of the disease. That is why we must prioritize good practices based on specific research, together with strong evidence on the multiple health benefits of regular and adequate amounts of physical activity in other cardio metabolic conditions, has led to physical inactivity be identified by national and international clinical practice guidelines as one of the multiple risk factors that require simultaneous intervention and principles for optimal prevention/management in rehabilitation. Despite this awareness, physical inactivity is not systematically addressed by the renal care teams from the care of the physiotherapist's professional in this section of the hemodialysis units [3].

Other disease conditions can accelerate the loss of kidney function as it is: diabetes, obesity, high blood pressure among others can cause dysfunction of multiple systems. [4, 5]. That is why physical activity at adequate levels and regularly prescribed allow positive contribution to the impact of muscle mass loss and weakness, low aerobic capacity, vascular reserve capacity, frailty and disability, where the latter are evidenced in a quality of life compromised in chronic kidney disease [6–10].

Among the changes resulting from chronic renal failure, muscle dysfunctions occur, where studies have shown the presence of atrophy of muscle fibers resulting from an imbalance between the synthesis and degradation of muscle protein. There may even be decreased synthesis and/or increased degradation [11–15]. Several mechanisms lead to muscle dysfunction, among which are: the depletion of amino acids; chronic inflammation; inactivity; malnutrition syndrome; changes in capillary perfusion; peripheral neuropathy, among others.

Thus, the literature reports exercise intolerance associated with anemia and hypervolemia in users with chronic renal failure; studies have already shown the treatment of these conditions, however, does not improve the tolerance to exercise, and therefore, this intolerance consequently leads to a sedentary lifestyle, which further decreases the physical capacity, creating a vicious circle within of the condition of chronic kidney disease translated into implications in their quality of life [16–18].

The foregoing evidences the need to complement the processes of renal rehabilitation with the clear participation of the physiotherapist as a promoter of the human body movement from the areas of secondary, tertiary prevention and rehabilitation with the aim of diminishing the negative impact of the burden of the disease in the user and carer.

1.1 Physiotherapy in the field of renal rehabilitation

The treatment of patients with progressive renal failure can be divided into several components, including health promotion and primary prevention programs (based on risk groups), early planning of renal replacement therapy and the establishment of interventions to treat the progression of chronic kidney disease and increase the quality of life of patients. Physiotherapy is included in this component of the treatment, based mainly on specific programs of supervised physical exercise, with the aim of increasing the level of physical fitness and, consequently, improving the quality of life and reducing the need for antihypertensive medications; morbidity and mortality [19].

The physiotherapeutic action in renal hemodialysis units is based on the prescription of their therapeutic actions based on physical activity, where it has been possible to demonstrate the benefits of physical activity for patients with chronic renal failure [20] including: increase in tolerance to exercise; reduction of inflammatory mediators; increase in synthesis and decrease in muscle protein degradation; increase in the number and size of muscle fibers, thus increasing muscle strength; increase in hematocrit and hemoglobin. Central effects also occur: improvement of left ventricular function, decrease in the occurrence of cardiac arrhythmias, in addition to beneficial effects on coronary artery disease risk factors (hypertension, lipid disorders).

Physical exercise is derived from the concept of physical activity, which is any movement of the body that spends energy above the basal level. Exercise then is all planned, structured and repetitive physical activity that aims to improve or maintain one or more components of physical condition. Therefore the prescription of physical exercise is the orderly and systematic process by which a regime of physical activity and/or exercise is recommended individually, according to needs and preferences, to obtain greater benefits with the lowest risk to health [21].

From this perspective, health professionals require a multidisciplinary work [22] that mainly involves physiotherapists [23] to counteract the progress of noncommunicable chronic diseases (NCD), using cost-effective actions that cover the entire population [24, 25].

1.2 Renal rehabilitation based on the strategy of the physical exercise in the unit of hemodialysis

The criteria for examination (anamnesis), evaluation and diagnosis, intervention processes, prognosis and evolution to contribute to the goals of the interdisciplinary group of renal rehabilitation at the hemodialysis units are set out in the process schema of the American Physiotherapy Practice Guide (APTA) [26].

The criteria for examination (anamnesis), evaluation and diagnosis, intervention processes, prognosis and evolution to contribute to the goals of the interdisciplinary group of renal rehabilitation are set out in the process schema of the American Physiotherapy Practice Guide (APTA).

Among the fundamental aspects in the process of the anamnesis with the user is the process of collecting important data for the development of the clinical history in physiotherapy as are the physical qualities that are immersed in the stay of hemodialysis units. Likewise, comorbidities, medications, postural changes, vital signs, and anthropometric data will be analyzed in order to evaluate the physical condition in health, to subsequently plan the prescription of the appropriate exercise according to the degree of severity of chronic kidney disease.

1.3 Contraindications and precautions in the physical exercise in the hemodialysis unit

Among the contraindications for the practice of physical activity prescribed by physiotherapy, some exclusion criteria are considered: recent myocardial infarction; uncontrolled arrhythmias; uncontrolled hypertension (systolic blood pressure > 200 mm Hg and diastolic blood pressure > 120 mm Hg); unstable angina; severe decompensated diabetes (blood glucose > 300 mg/dL); dysfunction of the left ventricle; presence of neurological or motor impeding dysfunction, for the application of the protocol of physical activity.

At the beginning of each exercise session, if the patient has any symptoms that prevent them from performing the exercises, the team of the hemodialysis unit should be informed, where they will report some important aspects such as: perceived muscle fatigue, angina pectoris, lipotimias, pallor, syncope, pre-syncope, disproportionate dyspnea in relation to intensity of effort, arrhythmias and hypotension or the hypertensive response of being detected any of these symptoms is important to study the admission to the physiotherapy program in hemodialysis within the rehabilitation program renal.

1.4 Effects of the physical exercise in renal rehabilitation

Patients with chronic kidney disease are inactive, which reduces physical performance. Aerobic exercise interventions have been shown to increase maximum oxygen consumption in selected patients. In addition, preliminary evidence, although mixed, suggests that aerobic exercise training may improve blood pressure, lipid profile, and mental health in this population.

The training with resistance exercises, although less studied, where an increase in muscular resistance and performance is observed, translates into an increase in functioning in their activities of daily life. Despite the evidence that exercise is safe and beneficial in patients with chronic kidney disease, dialysis patients remain inactive, where it is necessary to establish parameters from the evaluation, the advice of the physiotherapy intervention based on the physical exercise directed to the patients with this pathology.

The actions of physiotherapy are based on the evaluation of exercise capacity: measures of aerobic capacity assessment of exercise, muscle strength, and overall quality of life [27].

1.5 Muscular strength

The loss of muscle mass is the most important predictor of mortality in HD patients [28]. Muscular atrophy and, consequently, the organism is a generalized weakness, caused by the loss of strength, compared with normal subjects is 30–40% lower, making the patient physical deconditioning [29, 30]. Physical training is an important factor in the control and reversal of the loss, although the effects of this population have yet to be fully understood [31].

In this sense, Cantareli et al. [32] applied 5 months of resistance and strength training during HD, demonstrating the increase in muscle strength of the knee extensors and the average loads tolerated by MID: 4.71 ± 3.03 vs. 6.07 ± 2.62 vs. 8.42 ± 3.30 kg; MIE 4.85 ± 3.13 vs. 6.21 ± 2.82 vs. 8.57 ± 3.99 kg, $p < 0.05$. Other authors [33–36], studied the effect of aerobic and/or resistance also found a significant improvement in muscle strength.

Muscle fiber atrophy, type I and II, particularly type IIB, is an important factor that together with histochemical changes at low concentration of aerobic enzymes, low oxidative capacity, loss of capillarity and low levels of contractile proteins contribute to the muscle dysfunction [37, 38].

To verify the effects of exercise on the alterations present in patients with chronic renal failure in HD muscle, Sakkas et al. [12] examined the morphology of twin muscles in 12 patients before and after an aerobic exercise program performed three times a week for 6 months. The results showed that the proposed training improved muscle tropism, increased cross-sectional area by 46% and reduced the atrophy of muscle fibers of type I (51–15%), type IIA (5821%) and type IIB (62–32%). In addition, significant differences were found with respect to increased muscle capillarity.

Muscle strength is usually measured as maximal force by isokinetic dynamometry [39] and maximum torque, and absolute muscle strength using one maximum repetition [40] being the maximum weight that can be lifted in a single repetition of a given exercise by the physiotherapist.

1.6 Aerobic capacity

Several studies have shown that patients with chronic kidney disease on hemodialysis have reduced functional capacity and exercise capacity by about 50% lower compared to healthy subjects [41, 42]. Several factors associated with this reduction include decreased physical activity, muscle weakness, anemia, ventricular dysfunction, abnormal metabolic and hormonal controls [31]. Currently, great interest has been attributed to the assessment of the functional capacity of these patients through the six-minute walk test (PM6M) and other tests such as sitting and standing up. These tests are simple and measure functional capacity through basic information, and provide important data to monitor the progress of the patient in the course of the disease thus evaluating the benefits of rehabilitation programs [43].

1.7 Quality of life

Research has shown that chronic kidney disease and hemodialysis are some of the pathologies and therapies that most affect the quality of life, since they lead to the limitation of cardiorespiratory and physical capacity, which can degrade performance in work activities and social life [41, 44, 45]. Studies show that physical activity can contribute to an improvement in the quality of life of patients with chronic kidney disease.

Painter et al. [46] found the effect of a program consisting of 8 weeks of exercises at home, of 8 weeks of cycle ergometer during dialysis on the quality of life of chronic kidney patients. After 4 months, the authors observed a significant increase in the following dimensions of SF-36: functional capacity (47.7 ± 28.3 vs. 53.4 ± 27 $p = 0.004$), physical (40.4 ± 40, 3 vs. 54.5 ± 21.4 $p < 0.001$), pain (60.5 ± 28.1 vs. 66.6 ± 28.6 $p = 0.003$) and general health (45 ± 21.9 vs. 49, 1 ± 22.5 $p = 0.05$). According to the authors of the SF-36 results clearly indicate that specific physical activity affects the physical aspects of health, because there were no changes in mental health scores in any group of patients. Consequently, Vilsteren et al. [35] at 12 weeks of intra-dialysis aerobic training observed a significant change in the components of vitality and the general state from the application of the SF-36 questionnaire ($p = 0.001$).

However, Cantareli et al. [32] in his clinical trial of seven patients showed that the average values of the physical aspects, pain, general health and vitality increased after achieving an increase in muscle mass, but it was not very significant.

1.8 Existing barriers for participation in physical activity programs in renal units

Physical inactivity is a strong predictor of mortality in patients with end-stage renal disease and is associated with physical malfunction. Patients with terminal stage kidney disease are inactive even compared to sedentary individuals without kidney disease. Therefore, it is necessary to identify those existing barriers that have been described by some researches in hemodialysis units such as: Early muscular fatigue in the execution of movement, asthenia and adynamia, post-dialysis fatigue [47].

However, the lack of guidance from nephrologists is probably not the only reason for patient's low levels of physical activity. In a study by Goodman and colleagues [48], lack of motivation and interest were some of the factors cited as the limitation of the patient's participation in physical activity.

The deficit in physical activity among patients on dialysis has been theorized that it is due to a lack of motivation secondary to the patient's barriers, including socioeconomic, psychological and the perception of physical disability, although the motivation towards the practice and adherence of A physical activity program may be related to the previous level of physical exercise performed by the subject [49, 50].

However, given the potential obstacles to providing exercise opportunities in the dialysis unit, a possible alternative would be to promote health education mechanisms towards tertiary prevention aimed at users with the goal of identifying times in their daily routine (outside of dialysis) and thus incorporate physical activity effectively in their activities of daily life. Some guidance and encouragement should be guided by recommendations directed at older people from health professionals [51, 52].

2. Conclusions

Studies of the barriers to the participation of renal users in hemodialysis units where exercise programs are being carried out are needed.

It is also important to consolidate elements of the evaluation, recommendations from physiotherapy and its contribution to the rehabilitation program in order to continue on the path of evidence-based practice.

However, participants must be motivated to participate in moderate physical activity according to the current recommendations or consensus of the renal rehabilitation. Users who experience early fatigue or asthenia may benefit from strength training interventions, taking into account that aerobic and resistance exercises should be initiated at relatively low intensity in patients with this disease and progress taking into account the level of tolerance to exercise in order to avoid undesirable effects or even the suspension of therapeutic exercise.

Acknowledgements

The authors express their gratitude to the Manuela Beltrán University for its projection and interest in research topics in the field of kidney disease and human body movement.

Conflict of interest

The authors do not present conflicts of interest in the process of the narrative review type investigation.

Author details

Jorge Enrique Moreno Collazos* and Diana Carolina Zona Rubio
Cardiorespiratory Therapy Unit, Manuela Beltran University, Bogota, Colombia

*Address all correspondence to: jorge.moreno@docentes.umb.edu.co

References

[1] Farragher J, Jassal S. Rehabilitation of the geriatric dialysis patient. Seminars in Dialysis. 2012;**25**(6):649-656

[2] Evans M, Fryzek J, Elinder CG, et al. The natural history of chronic renal failure: Results from an unselected, population-based, inception cohort in Sweden. American Journal of Kidney Diseases. 2006;**46**:863-870

[3] Koufaki P, Greenwood S, Painter P, Mercer T. The BASES expert statement on exercise therapy for people with chronic kidney disease. Journal of Sports Sciences. 2015;**33**(18):1902-1907

[4] Tentori F, Elder S, Robinson B, et al. Physical exercise among participants in the dialysis outcomes and practice patterns study [DOPPS]: Correlates and associated outcomes. Nephrology, Dialysis, Transplantation: Official Publication of the European Dialysis and Transplant Association-European Renal Association. 2010;**25**(9):3050-3062

[5] Smart N, Steele M. Exercise training in haemodialysis patients: A systematic review and meta-analysis. Nephrology. 2011;**16**(7):626-632

[6] Segura-Ortí E. Exercise in haemodyalisis patients: A literature systematic review. Nefrología: Publicación Oficial de la Sociedad Española Nefrologia. 2010;**30**(2):236-246

[7] Koufaki P, Kouidi E. Current best evidence recommendations on measurement and interpretation of physical function in patients with chronic kidney disease. Sports Medicine. 2010;(12):1055

[8] Phan K, Jia F, Kamper SJ. Effects of regular physical exercise training in adults with chronic kidney disease. British Journal of Sports Medicine. 2016;**50**(5):317-318

[9] Smart N, Williams A, Fassett R, et al. Review: Exercise & Sports Science Australia [ESSA] position statement on exercise and chronic kidney disease. Journal of Science and Medicine in Sport. 2013;**16**:406-411

[10] Heiwe S, Jacobson S. Original investigation: Exercise training in adults with CKD: A systematic review and meta-analysis. American Journal of Kidney Diseases. 2014;**64**:383-393

[11] Bohannon RW, Smith J, Hull D, Palmeri D, Barnhard R. Deficits in lower extremity muscle and gait performance among transplant kidney candidates. Archives of Physical Medicine and Rehabilitation. 1995;**76**(6):547-551

[12] Sakkas GK, Sargeant AJ, Mercer TH, Ball D, Koufaki P, Karatzaferi C, et al. Changes in muscle morphology in dialysis patients after 6 months of aerobic exercise training. Nephrology, Dialysis, Transplantation. 2003;**18**(9):1854-1861

[13] Kosmadakis GC, Bevington A, Smith AC, Clapp EL, Viana JL, Bishop NC, et al. Physical exercise in patients with severe kidney disease. Nephron. Clinical Practice. 2010;**115**(1):c7-c16

[14] Adams GR, Vaziri ND. Skeletal muscle dysfunction in chronic renal failure: Effects of exercise. American Journal of Physiology. Renal Physiology. 2006;**290**(4):F753-F761

[15] Hopman WM, Harrison MB, Coo H, Friedberg E, Buchanan M, VanDenKerkhof EG. Associations between chronic disease, age and physical and mental health status. Chronic Diseases in Canada. 2009;**29**(2):108-116

[16] Carvalho T. Diretriz de reabilitação cardiopulmonar e metabólica: Aspectos práticos e responsabilidades.

Arquivos Brasileiros de Cardiologia. 2006;**86**(1):74-82

[17] Martins MRI, Cesarino CB. Quality of life in chronic kidney failure patients receiving hemodialysis treatment. Revista Latino-Americana de Enfermagem. 2005;**13**(5):670-676

[18] Reboredo MM, Henrique DMN, Bastos MG, Paula RB. Exercício físico em pacientes dialisados. Revista Brasileira de Medicina do Esporte. 2007;**13**(6):427-430

[19] Miranda G, Souza B, Oliveira F. Impact of physical therapy on functional capacity and life quality of patients with chronic kidney disease/ Impacto da fisioterapia na qualidade de vida e capacidade funcional em pacientes com doença renal crônica. Fisioterapia Em Movimento. 2014;(4):643

[20] Nascimento LCA, Coutinho EB, Silva KNG. Effectiveness of physical exercise in chronic renal failure. Fisioterapia e Pesquisa. 2012;**25**(1):231-239

[21] Fortier M, Tulloch H, Hogg W. A good fit integrating physical activity counselors into family practice. Canadian Family Physician. 2006;**52**(8):942-944

[22] Moore GE. The role of exercise prescription in chronic disease. British Journal of Sports Medicine. 2004;**38**(1):6-7

[23] Quality Assurance Agency for Higher Education. Benchmark Statement: Health Care Programmes. Phase 1: Physiotherapy. London: Frontier Print & Design Limited; 2001

[24] WCPT. European Core Standards of Physiotherapy Practice General Meeting of the European Region of the WCPT; Athens: WCPT; 2008. pp. 1-46

[25] De Vries TP, Henning RH, Hogerzeil HG, Fresle DA. El proceso de la terapéutica razonada. En: Guía de la Buena Prescripción. Barcelona: OMS; 1998. pp. 6-12

[26] Task Force for the Development of Student Clinical Performance Instruments. The development and testing of APTA clinical performance instruments. American Physical Therapy Association. Physical Therapy. 2002;**82**(4):329

[27] Johansen KL. Exercise and chronic kidney disease. Sports Medicine. 2005;**35**(6):485-499

[28] Cheema BS, Smith BC, Singh MA. A rationale for intradialytic exercise training as standard clinical practice in ESRD. American Journal of Kidney Diseases. 2005;**45**(5):912-916

[29] Soares A, Zehetmeyer M, Rabuske M. Atuação da fisioterapia durante a hemodiálise visando à qualidade de vida do paciente renal crônico. Revista de Saúde da Universidade Católica de Pelotas. 2007;**1**(1):7-12

[30] Medeiros RH, Pinent CEC, Meyer F. Aptidão física de indivíduo com doença renal crônica. Jornal Brasileiro de Nefrologia. 2002;**24**(2):81-87

[31] Coelho DM, Ribeiro JM, Soares DD. Exercícios físicos durante a hemodiálise: uma revisão sistemática. Jornal Brasileiro de Nefrologia. 2008;**30**(2):88-98

[32] Cantareli F, Corrêa LB, Oliveira RN, Cunha LS. Efeito do treinamento muscular periférico na capacidade funcional e qualidade de vida nos pacientes em hemodiálise. Jornal Brasileiro de Nefrologia. 2009;**31**(1):18-24

[33] Storer TW, Casaburi R, Sawelson S, Kopple JD. Endurance exercise training during haemodialysis

improves strength, power, fatigability and physical performance in maintenance haemodialysis patients. Nephrology, Dialysis, Transplantation. 2005;**20**(1):429-437

[34] Cheema B, Abas H, Smith B, O'Sullivan A, Chan M, Patwardhan A, et al. Progressive exercise training for anabolism in kidney disease [PEAK]: A randomized, controlled trial of resistance training during hemodialysis. Journal of the American Society of Nephrology. 2007;**18**(15):94-601

[35] Vilsteren MCBA, Greef MHG, Huisman RM. The effects of a low-to-moderate intensity pre-conditioning exercise programme linked with exercise counseling for sedentary haemodialysis patients in the Netherlands: Results of a randomized clinical trial. Nephrology, Dialysis, Transplantation. 2005;**20**(1):141-146

[36] Molsted S, Eidemakb I, Sorensena HT, Kristensen JH. Five months of physical exercise in hemodialysis patients: Effects on aerobic capacity, physical function and self-rated health. Nephron. Clinical Practice. 2004;**96**(3):c76-c81

[37] Moreira PR, Barros E. Atualização em fisiologia e fisiopatologia renal: Bases fisiopatológicas da miopatia na insuficiência renal crônica. Jornal Brasileiro de Nefrologia. 2000;**22**(1):40-44

[38] Coelho MC, Godoy CG, Tavares H, Navarro F, Almeida AL. Avaliação funcional e prescrição de treinamento para paciente portador de insuficiência renal crônica submetido a hemodiálise: Um relato de caso. Revista Brasileira de Prescrição e Fisiologia do Exercício. 2007;**1**(3):29-41

[39] Kouidi E, Albani M, Konstantinos N. The effects of exercise training on muscle atrophy in haemodialysis patients. Nephrology, Dialysis, Transplantation. 1998;**13**:685-699

[40] Heiwe S, Clyne N, Tollback A, Borg K. Effects of regular resistance training on muscle histopathology and morphometry in elderly patients with chronic kidney disease. American Journal of Physical Medicine & Rehabilitation. 2005;**84**:865-874

[41] Cunha MS, Andrade V, Guedes CAV, Meneghetti CHZ, Aguiar AP, Cardoso AL. Avaliação da capacidade funcional e da qualidade de vida em pacientes renais crônicos submetidos a tratamento hemodialítico. Fisioterapia e Pesquisa. 2009;**16**(2):155-160

[42] Jatobá JPC, Amaro WF, Andrade APA, Cardoso FPF, Monteiro AMH, Oliveira MAM. Avaliação da função pulmonar, força muscular respiratória e teste de caminhada de seis minutos em pacientes portadores de doença renal crônica em hemodiálise. Jornal Brasileiro de Nefrologia. 2008;**30**(4):280-287

[43] Cury JL, Brunetto AF, Aydos RD. Efeitos negativos da insuficiência renal crônica sobre a função pulmonar e a capacidade funcional. Revista Brasileira de Fisioterapia. 2010;**14**(2):91-98

[44] Barbosa LMM, Andrade MP Jr, Bastos KA. Preditores de qualidade de vida em pacientes com doença renal crônica em hemodiálise. Jornal Brasileiro de Nefrologia. 2007;**29**(4):222-229

[45] Castro M, Caiuby AVS, Draibe A, Canziani ME. Qualidade de vida de pacientes com insuficiência renal crônica em Hemodiálise avaliada através do instrumento genérico SF-36. Revista da Associação Médica Brasileira. 2003;**49**(3):245-249

[46] Painter P, Carlson L, Carey S, Paul SM, Myll J. Physical functioning and

health related quality-of-life changes with exercise training in hemodialysis patients. American Journal of Kidney Diseases. 2000;**35**(3):482-492

[47] Jafarzadeh Esfehani A, Dashti S. Barriers to exercise participation among dialysis patients. Nephrology, Dialysis, Transplantation. 2012;**27**(10):3964-3964

[48] Goodman ED, Ballou MB. Perceived barriers and motivators to exercise in hemodialysis patients. Nephrology Nursing Journal. 2004;**31**:23-29

[49] King AC, Castro C, Wilcox S, et al. Personal and environmental factors associated with physical inactivity among different racial ethnic groups of U.S. middle-aged and older-aged women. Health Psychology. 2000;**19**:354-364

[50] Delgado C, Johansen KL. Deficient counseling on physical activity among nephrologists. Nephron. Clinical Practice. 2010;**116**:330-336

[51] Bennett PN, Breugelmans L, Barnard R, et al. Sustaining a hemodialysis exercise program: A review. Seminars in Dialysis. 2010;**23**:62-73

[52] Pianta TF. The role of physical therapy in improving physical functioning of renal patients. Advances in Renal Replacement Therapy. 1999;**6**:149-158